D0952534

# WHY DIRT IS GOOD

5 WAYS TO MAKE
GERMS YOUR FRIENDS

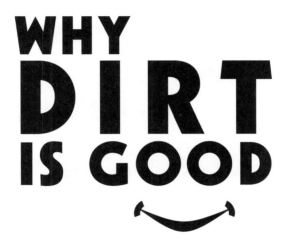

WHY
DIRT
IS GOOD

MARY RUEBUSH, PhD

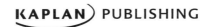

**KAPLAN** PUBLISHING

Published by Kaplan Publishing, a division of Kaplan, Inc.
1 Liberty Plaza, 24th Floor
New York, NY 10006

Printed in the United States of America

Library of Congress Cataloging-in-Publication Data

Ruebush, Mary.
  Why dirt is good : 5 ways to make germs your friends / Mary Ruebush.
    p. cm.
  ISBN 978-1-4277-9804-6
  1. Immune system. 2. Immunity. 3. Bacteria. 4. Viruses.
  5. Microbiology. I. Title.
  QR181.R84 2009
  616.07'9--dc22

                                      2008042683

10 9 8 7 6 5 4 3 2 1

ISBN-13: 978-1-4277-9804-6

Kaplan Publishing books are available at special quantity discounts to use for sales promotions, employee premiums, or educational purposes. Please email our Special Sales Department to order or for more information at kaplanpublishing@kaplan.com, or write to Kaplan Publishing, 1 Liberty Plaza, 24th Floor, New York, NY 10006.

# Contents

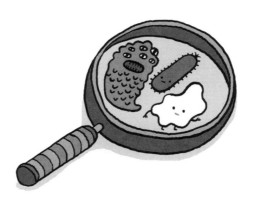

# Introduction

In your bag, under your sink, and on your desk, they're everywhere: antibacterial sprays and hand sanitizers. We arm ourselves with weapons against the unseen threat of dirty microbes. But if we win the war on germs, humankind could be the final casualty. What we need today isn't less dirt, it's more.

We certainly understand more about sanitation and medicine than we did 50 years ago, and yet we seem to be trading old plagues for new ones. With our standards of national cleanliness so much improved, why do we see increasing rates of asthma, childhood diabetes, and many other autoimmune diseases, to say nothing of a dangerous rise in antibiotic-resistant germs?

The more we hear about new diseases, the more we spend on chemicals to "sterilize" our environments. At the slightest hint of personal discomfort, we run for the drugstore to refill our prescriptions. What we accomplish by this behavior is definitely not what is best for the human race. Our short-term fixes are weakening our own natural immunity and strengthening the disease agents that attack us. We are raising a new generation of "superbugs" that are impossible to treat.

The human immune system is a miracle of millennia of evolution. What is needed now is a simple return to common sense—the idea of letting Mother Nature take her course.

If you understand the grand design of the immune system, it becomes obvious that your immune response is just another body part that needs exercise to become strong. And as in so many other cases, healthy choices we make in childhood prepare us to run the marathon of life. What you need to do to protect yourself and your family may surprise you: Let them eat dirt, and avoid antibiotics whenever possible.

As a microbiology and immunology teacher at the medical school level and a mother of two, I know a lot about germs. In *Why Dirt Is Good*, I introduce you to your immune system and tell you how it fights germs. I then share the five rules I've distilled from my decades of study. These five rules are crucial for helping you to lead a long and healthy life. They're simple and easy to follow:

- Rule 1: Let them eat dirt. Exposure to dirt helps children build strong immune systems that will provide lifelong protection.

- Rule 2. Use it or lose it. To work as well as possible, your immune system needs exercise just as the rest of you does.

- Rule 3: Don't encourage superbugs. Avoid antimicrobics such as antibacterial soap and antibiotic drugs whenever possible.

- Rule 4: Keep your vaccinations up to date. Vaccines give you safe, effective immunity the easy way.

- Rule 5. Always ask first, what would Mother Nature do? Common sense is the best cure for most infections. Save drugs for when they're really needed.

Parents of messy kids beware: Habits your mother always told you to avoid (like chewing your nails) actually do strengthen your immune system. Prepare to have your beliefs about dirt challenged!

- - - - - - - - - - - - - - -

# PART ONE

# How Your Immune System Works

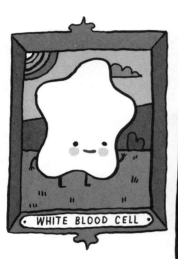

WHITE BLOOD CELL

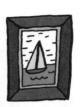

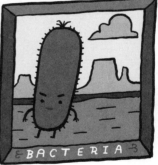

BACTERIA

# Meet Your Immune System

To read the news headlines or to watch any TV commercials, you'd think that the only thing standing between you and death by some horrible new disease such as Ebola fever is the germ-killing power of some miraculous cleaning product. Actually, what keeps most people healthy most of the time is the amazing ability of your body to keep infection out to begin with, and to deal with it efficiently if it does manage to enter your body. All that cleaning doesn't protect you nearly as well as your own body can.

Your immune system begins with the physical barriers that keep dangerous germs out of your body. These are your first line of defense against invaders. The most obvious of these barriers is your skin itself. The largest organ in your body (the average adult's skin covers about 20 square feet), your skin wraps your entire body in a tough, flexible, waterproof covering designed to keep microorganisms out and moisture in.

Wherever your skin joins the openings into your body, such as your nose or mouth, mucosal surfaces take over. Mucosal surfaces secrete mucus, a thick slimy substance we all know and love, whose role is to coat potential invaders and slide them out of the body. Mucosal surfaces are made up of epithelial cells, flat cells that fit together tightly, sort of like shingles. They line your respiratory tract, your digestive tract, and your reproductive tract from end to end. In your respiratory tract, for instance, the mucosal surfaces are very good at trapping microorganisms and sending them back out of your body through sneezing or coughing. In your digestive tract, microorganisms are eliminated in the feces.

Your body also has chemical defenses. The strong acid in your stomach and small intestine kills many microorganisms before they can even get as far as trying to penetrate the cells that line your digestive tract. Even your eyes form a defense — tears wash away microorganisms. Both tears and saliva contain antibacterial compounds that protect those areas of your body from invaders.

## Beyond Barriers

All the physical and chemical barriers to infection work together to keep harmful microbes out of your body. Even so, plenty still manage to get in. If that's the case, why aren't you sick all the time? Put another way, what keeps you mostly healthy most of the time?

It's your immune system — the amazingly complex, intricate, and efficient protective army Mother Nature has evolved for us over millions of years. Your immune system is made up of different types of cells that circulate everywhere throughout your body, constantly patrolling for invaders and attacking them when they're found. All those different cell types work together in a highly coordinated way to protect you from invaders—no one type of cell can do the whole job of finding and killing a germ, much less remembering that particular germ for the rest of your life.

It takes all the cell types of your immune system, working together, to do that. Just as it takes all the different systems of your car—the transmission, the cooling system, the fuel system, the brakes, and so on—working together to make the car run properly, all the different parts of your immune system need to work together as well. So, even though your immune system is really one big, complicated, and interconnected system, we can get a good idea of how it works by breaking it down into its separate parts.

## The Cells of Your Immune System

The cells that make up your immune system are generically called white blood cells. Actually, they're not white—they're clear and colorless. They're called white blood cells to distinguish them from the red blood cells, which get their color from hemoglobin, the chemical that binds oxygen and carries it within the cell. Platelets, the tiny blood cells that are used for clotting, are also red.

You have a number of different types of white blood cells, each having a very specific function within the immune system. They fall into two main groups, depending on how they arise within your body.

All your white blood cells (and red blood cells, too) are made in your bone marrow, especially in the long bones of your arms and legs. Every single blood cell in your system, regardless of type, starts out in your bone marrow as a stem cell — the most basic sort of cell in your body. Stem cells in your bone marrow have the potential to become any one of the many different types of blood cells, red and white, by following one of two possible paths. Along one path, the stem cell develops into a cell that becomes a red blood cell or one of the types of white blood cells that make up your innate immune system. The other path is a little more targeted: These stem cells develop into cells that become the cells of your adaptive immune system.

Your immune system has two arms — the innate system and the adaptive system — and although both arms have to work in tandem to keep you healthy, they each have different roles to play — roles that need different kinds of white blood cells.

## Innate Immunity

Let's start with the innate immune system. This is the system that kicks in the moment your barrier defenses are breached by an intruder — when you scrape a knuckle, for instance. The white blood cells that immediately come to the rescue fall into two basic categories: eaters and flamethrowers. More scientifically, cells that eat invaders and debris in the body are called phagocytes, from the Greek word *phage* meaning to devour. These have three basic types: monocytes (immature macrophages that circulate in the bloodstream), macrophages (literally, "big eaters"), and neutrophils.

# Handy Guide to Your White Blood Cells, or Your Body's Cellular Army

| System | White Blood Cell Type | Function |
|---|---|---|
| **Innate Immunity** | Monocyte | Circulates in your blood until needed in the tissues; then exits the bloodstream and becomes a macrophage |
| | Macrophage | The big eater—destroys invaders by engulfing and digesting them. Helps to activate T cells |
| | Neutrophil | The most abundant white blood cell in your body. Circulates in the blood until needed in the tissues, then exits the bloodstream and destroys invaders by eating and digesting them. When this cell is frustrated by too much to eat it becomes bulimic and sterilizes the area with its "vomit" |
| | Mast cell | Granulocytic or flamethrower cell that fights parasites and is involved in allergic reactions |
| | Eosinophil | Granulocytic or flamethrower cell that fights parasites and is involved in allergic reactions |

*cont'd on next page*

| System | White Blood Cell Type | Function |
|---|---|---|
| | Basophil | Granulocytic or flamethrower cell that fights parasites and is involved in allergic reactions |
| | Natural killer cell | Cell that destroys a variety of invaders, including bacteria, viruses, tumor cells, fungi, and parasites. Abbreviated as NK |
| **Adaptive Immunity** | B cell | Antibody-producing cells |
| | T cell | Cells that control the immune response |
| | Helper T cell | A type of T cell that produces chemical signals to activate and direct the immune response. Abbreviated as Th |
| | Killer T cell | T cells that directly attack and destroy cells infected with viruses or changed by cancer processes. Also called a cytotoxic T lymphocyte (CTL) |

Macrophages live in the spaces between your cells. (Your body may seem very solid to you, but at the cellular level it's actually pretty porous; macrophages can easily slip between the cells.) As they move around your body, macrophages engulf and gobble up the dead cells and cellular debris that are a natural part of your body's normal processes. They're also on the lookout for any microorganism that may have gotten past the barrier systems.

Neutrophils circulate in your bloodstream. They're the most abundant type of white blood cell in your body. They're also the kamikaze soldiers of your immune system. When they're needed at a particular point in your body, they charge out of the bloodstream and go directly to the infected area. Like macrophages, they gobble up invaders, but they get "full" quickly. No problem — the neutrophils become bulimic and vomit up the digested bits of the invader and their own acidic contents. Neutrophils basically eat until they explode.

Granulocytes are cells that dump granules of toxic chemicals on invaders as a way of not-so-gently encouraging them to leave your body. These have four basic types: neutrophils, basophils, mast cells, and eosinophils. Neutrophils eat invaders, and also start the extracellular digestion process using toxic granules. Basophils (and mast cells that develop from them) and eosinophils are important for defense against worms and other parasites, and play a big role in allergic reactions. On the other hand, eosinophils also eat invaders, so in that sense they can be considered phagocytes—which all goes to show that the parts of the immune system interconnect and don't fit neatly into compartments.

Natural killer cells are another important part of your innate immune system. Although natural killer cells (abbreviated as NK) don't arise from the type of stem cell that produces the other cells of the innate immune system, they function as part of it. NK cells work in two ways. First, they can sense when your macrophages are at work attacking invaders. When they do, they secrete chemicals that stimulate the macrophages to work even harder. Second, NK cells can kill directly by binding to an invader and basically telling it to commit suicide. NK cells are important for defending you against viruses, which enter inside your cells to reproduce. They're also important for protecting you against some forms of cancer. They don't play much of a role in defending against other invaders, such as bacteria, that stay in between your cells, not inside them.

Your innate immune system also has another part that doesn't involve white blood cells at all. It's called your complement system, and it consists of some 25 or so different proteins that are made in your liver and float around in large quantities in your blood. They assist your immune cells. When the complement proteins sense the presence of alien proteins from an invading bacterium, they assemble through a complex chemical chain reaction. When the reaction is complete, the complement proteins have put themselves together into a chemical drill bit that bores a hole into the germ. A hole in its wall is not a good thing for a germ. The invader dies by filling up with fluid that leaks in from the surrounding tissue and exploding, or by being captured and eaten by a macrophage before it gets a chance to blow up.

## Adaptive Immunity

As your innate immune system fends off the invader, it also calls for help from the second line of defense, your adaptive immune system. The white blood cells of the adaptive arm are called lymphocytes. They don't eat germs or fire flamethrowers. Instead, they target and direct.

The cells of adaptive immunity fall into two categories: B cells and T cells. These cells are a bit smarter than the innate immune system cells. They can recognize specific attackers and then multiply wildly to produce the weapons that will destroy them. They also regulate the action of other white blood cells and kill infected cells within your body.

B cells get their name because they are born and "educated" within the bone marrow (B for bone). B cells learn their job—how to recognize a specific invader and target it for destruction—while nestled inside the bone marrow. From there, they venture out into your body, ready to put their home-schooled education to work. B cells make antibodies, which are proteins that seek out antigens on the surface of the invader.

What's an antigen? It's anything that makes your immune system cells react. Usually an antigen is a specific molecule found on the surface of a bacterium or other invader. Every type of germ has its own particular antigen that sets it apart from every other type of germ. Amazingly, your body can produce antibodies to every conceivable type of antigen.

Like a key in a lock, antibodies latch on to the antigens, clogging up the membrane of the cell and tagging it for quick destruction by complement proteins and phagocytes.

T cells start out in your bone marrow, just like B cells, but when it comes time for their education, they go away to school. They leave the bone marrow and end up in your thymus (hence T), an organ in your chest. While they're in the thymus, T cells can go down one of two paths. One path turns them into helper T cells, cells that will direct and control the immune response. The other turns them into killer T cells, cells that can directly kill invaders. Like B cells, T cells have receptors that can recognize virtually any invader. Once these receptors are activated, helper T cells take over the immune system response—you could think of them as the general directing the overall battle, or the coach directing the game. The helper Ts send out chemical messenger signals to the other immune cells that coordinate and amplify the attack. Some of those signals tell B cells to get to work producing antibodies, while others stimulate more eater cells (macrophages and neutrophils) to go to the site of the infection and make them eat even faster. Helper T cells also send out signals that tell killer T cells to seek out and destroy infected cells.

When the battle is over, some of those helper T cells remember what happened for the rest of your life. The next time the same invader tries to attack, the T cells will respond almost instantly and demolish them. The same is true for B cells. After the invaders have all been ousted, your B cells remember them—forever. The next time they try to attack, the B cells remember exactly which antibody worked the last time and immediately start making it again.

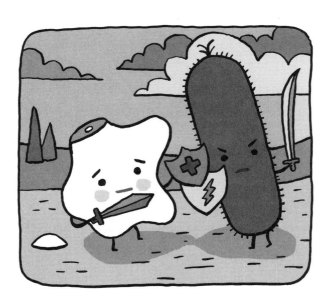

# You versus Germs

You need all those immune defenses I've just described because your body is under constant attack by germs. They lurk on elevator buttons and on shopping cart handles. They travel through coughs and sneezes by your coworkers and your kids. What we call germs are microorganisms of all sorts, but especially harmful bacteria, viruses, fungi, and parasites. But does being under constant attack mean you're going to get sick all the time? Of course not.

Here's a major reason dirt is good: Your immune system has been exquisitely fine tuned by millions of years of evolution to let you live in balance, more or less, with all the many dangerous microorganisms that are out there. But to do that, your immune system needs to be exposed to germs to build your ability to produce the right response quickly. If you somehow were raised in a sterile environment where all harmful germs were eliminated, your immune system wouldn't ever get activated. If you then had to leave your sterile environment to join the real world, you'd be an easy target for any germ that came along, because your immune system would be very slow to respond correctly.

Why do all those germs want to get into you? Because inside, you're nicely warm and wet, with a good supply of nutrients—exactly what a germ needs to thrive and multiply.

Not every germ is dangerous. Right now, as you read this, even if you just took a shower and washed with antimicrobial soap, the outside of your body teems with literally trillions of microbes—bacteria, viruses, fungi, and assorted parasites. On the inside, you're just one big microbe ranch. Inside your mouth alone are some six hundred bacterial species; there are hundreds of millions of bacteria in every drop of your saliva. In all, the typical human probably harbors some 90 trillion microbes, outnumbering the cells of your body by about 10 to one. For the most part, our bodies have evolved to coexist with the germs around us, even the harmful ones. We all carry around a massive load of microbes. It's called our normal flora.

Eons of evolution have adapted your body to coexist with all those microbes. Paradoxically, the very fact that you have so many microbes of so many different kinds is what keeps you healthy most of the time. All those different microbes are competing with each other to take up residence in some part of your body. Most of the prime real estate in your body, like your skin or gums, is taken up by bacteria that are either harmless or even helpful. In the endless, fierce competition for space, there's not much room for the minority of bacteria that are dangerous to humans. They generally can't get enough of a foothold to start reproducing fast enough to outpace the normal flora. Not only that—normal flora fight back.

Many species of *Streptococcus* bacteria live in your mouth, for instance. Not all strep bacteria are harmful, though, and in fact you want to have a good range of strep species in your mouth. That's because some of them give off chemicals that inhibit the growth of two well-known bad actors among the streps: *Streptococcus pyogenes* (this one gives you "strep throat") and *S. pneumoniae* (as the name suggests, this one gives you pneumonia). If the bad streps can't get a solid foothold within the vast crowd of all the other bacteria, they can't do any harm.

As another example, intestinal bacteria help digest your food and even produce some of the vitamins you need. Without the K vitamins provided by our normal intestinal flora, for example, we would all bleed to death from an inability to produce the clotting necessary to stop bleeding.

But what about the bad guys? To understand what Mother Nature has devised as her answer to all the various types of infections that can attack you at any moment, it's important to understand a little something about the categories of disease agents.

The smallest invaders of your body are viruses. These organisms are extremely small. How small? A red blood cell has a diameter of six to eight microns—and a micron is a millionth of a meter. About a thousand viruses would fit inside a red blood cell, and about 20 bacteria would fit inside a red blood cell. Conversely, fungi are about 1.5 times the size of a red blood cell, and parasites start at about three times the size of a red blood cell. A virus is really just some genetic material (DNA or RNA) wrapped in a protein coating, making it about as small as an organism can be. Viruses are totally parasitic on your cells. To live and reproduce, a virus has to enter a cell and then "hijack" its normal function to complete its own life cycle. Once a virus enters your body, it immediately starts hunting for a cell to hijack.

Different viruses infect different cells. Cold viruses like the cells that line your respiratory tract, while diarrheal viruses like the cells of your intestines, because those cells have receptors on their surfaces that are complementary to the surface of the virus. Once a virus finds a cell it likes, it gets busy with the business of making baby viruses. Some viruses, such as most cold viruses, multiply wildly, swell up your cells, and make them burst to release the next generation of viruses. Other viruses, such as the human immunodeficiency virus (HIV) and some viruses associated with causing cancer, keep cells alive and bud off their surfaces slowly to release their babies.

Bacteria are a category of germs that are larger than viruses. They're still considerably smaller than your immune cells, which means that phagocytes can easily engulf and digest them. Bacteria have an edge over phagocytes, however: They can multiply extremely fast, so fast that they may often simply overwhelm the ability of your phagocytes to eat them all. That's one reason your body's ability to form an abscess is so important to your immune defenses. Those bacteria that can't be eaten quickly can still be walled off and killed by bulimic neutrophils and by the other cells of the immune system.

# How Your Immune System Defends You

Once a harmful germ manages to breach your outer defenses by getting through your skin or mucosal surfaces, your immune system immediately goes into action. Let's say you gash your finger with your garden clippers. Your first response is to swear loudly. Your immune system's first response is inflammation.

Any breach of your body's external barriers, such as a cut, lets germs enter and start multiplying. Your body's response is almost instantaneous: The germs must die. So, when your cut finger comes under attack from a bad germ that got carried in by the clipper blade, the first thing you're likely to notice is inflammation: The area around the cut becomes red, swollen, hot, and painful. What's happening is that the blood vessels nearest the infected area get a little swollen and "leaky," which allows white blood cells to enter the area more easily. The area swells up with blood, fluid, and white blood cells, all of which provide outward pressure.

The pressure pushes invaders out of your tissues, or at least keeps them from penetrating any farther inward. The rush of fluid and increased blood flow to the area also cause the other classic symptoms of inflammation: redness, heat, and pain.

Inflammation is an automatic response to injuries and illness. No matter how you manage to hurt yourself, and no matter what invader manages to get in, white blood cells will rush out of the bloodstream and into the area in response. Inflammation plays several critical roles in protecting you. First, it brings in the phagocytes, which will attempt to eat any invader and wall off the area from further invasion. Second, it increases blood flow into the area and makes the blood vessels in the area a little leaky. That carries in more white blood cells and lets them escape out of the bloodstream and into the tissue more easily.

Inflammation's effects aren't limited to the immune system. In the case of your cut finger, for instance, the swelling also brings in other substances, such as platelets to clot the blood, which will begin the healing process.

## What Is Dirt?

Germs are everywhere: around us, on us, in us. I use the word *dirt* in this book as a sort of shorthand for all the various ways we come into contact with all those germs. That obviously means soil, because humus, the organic part of soil, is crammed with bacteria, fungi, protozoa, and even viruses. It also means all the other germ-laden things we normally encounter, such as raw foods, and all the germ-laden places we go, like public bathrooms and kindergarten classrooms. Because our bodies are well adapted to handle a certain level of dirt, too much cleanliness can actually be harmful. The reasons dirt is good are many, as this book explains. That doesn't mean I think we should live in filth, drink contaminated water, eat contaminated food, and so on, all in the name of exercising our immune systems.

Starting in the 1870s and 1880s, public health measures in American cities brought clean water, regular garbage collection, public bathhouses, and other sanitation steps to their residents. The incidence of dangerous diseases such as cholera and typhoid dropped markedly, definitely a good thing. Today most of us live at a high level of public cleanliness — our water and food supplies are very safe, our trash is hauled away, and widespread vaccination and public health measures have virtually eliminated many of the infectious

*cont'd on next page*

diseases that killed so many a century ago. After well over a century of battling successfully against germs, we have the idea that if pretty good cleanliness is good, then supergood cleanliness is even better. Supergood cleanliness has started to backfire badly on us. As this book is meant to explain, for good health what we need is more dirt, not less, in our lives.

Once the inflammatory process is launched, your macrophages and neutrophils go into action. Since the most likely place to encounter an invader who makes it through a barrier is just past the barrier, macrophages particularly like to hang out just below the surface of your skin and just below the surface of the epithelial cells — in your throat, for instance. Most of the time they have a leisurely life, cleaning up bits of debris from your own cells. But when they encounter an invader, they get annoyed. Macrophages are already the largest of your immune system cells — they're about twice the size of T or B cells. Angry macrophages immediately start engulfing and digesting as many invaders as they can catch and start getting even bigger. At the same time, the macrophages send out a help signal calling for backup.

The first responders to the emergency signal are neutrophils, which are the most numerous and aggressive white blood cells in your body (they make up about 70 percent of your white blood cells). Neutrophils are the foot soldiers of your immune system. They flood into the area from the bloodstream and launch a kamikaze attack on the invader. They eat as much as they can, gorging themselves on both the invading bacteria and the debris of your own injured cells. When they can't eat any more, they become bulimic and start ejecting the digested bits out into the infected area. Neutrophils are expendable — they eat until they can't eat any more, then they blow up. The substance the neutrophils eject is acidic and helps to clean up the area of infection, though it may not seem that way to you when you look at the red, oozing cut on your finger. The result of the kamikaze attack is pus: the liquefied debris of dead and dying bacteria and dead and dying cells. This is what causes boils, pimples, styes — what doctors call an abscess.

While an abscess might be unsightly, annoying, and even painful, it's also a sign that your immune system is hard at work.

When you're sick with something like a cold, your immune system's first response is inflammation as well. It's more generalized than when you cut your finger, but your red, swollen nose, fever, and sore throat are all signs of inflammation.

The macrophages and neutrophils are in a race against the invader. Bacteria can multiply very rapidly, producing a new generation in just minutes. Many harmful bacteria also give off dangerous toxins that cause many of the symptoms of illness, such as diarrhea from salmonellosis. Bacteria live in your body in the spaces in between cells, where macrophages and neutrophils can find and eat them easily.

Viruses, however, bore their way into your cells and take them over, using your own cells to reproduce themselves. Reproduce they do, in large numbers. When the baby viruses burst out of the cell to find new cells to infect, the host cell dies.

Because it can take several days or even longer for your T and B cells to be fully activated, the macrophages and neutrophils hold the fort against the infection while the adaptive immune system cells work behind the lines to organize a major offensive.

While they're busy fighting the infection, macrophages also send help messages to your T cells, telling them to start organizing their attack. To understand how this works, think of macrophages as very messy eaters who have burped up crumbs of their meal and now have the crumbs (actually, bits of protein from the invader) stuck on them. Some of these macrophages leave the infected area and head to the nearest lymph node, taking their crumbs with them. They're looking for T cells, and the nearest lymph node is the quickest way to find them.

Your lymph nodes are small, bean-shaped structures that filter and recirculate lymph, the clear fluid that bathes the intercellular spaces of your body. You have about five to six hundred lymph nodes in your body; clusters of them are found in the underarms, neck, chest, abdomen, and groin. To your B and T cells, lymph nodes are like dating bars. They hang out in them, waiting to meet up with a germ carrying their counterpart antigens — molecular particles that identify a germ as a germ. Every one of your B and T cells has antigen receptor molecules on its surface. The receptor molecules are different on almost every cell — only a handful of each type of cell will have the same receptor. Since you have many millions of B and T cells, that means you have B and T cells with receptors that are specific for any possible invader you may encounter in your life. When a cell with the right receptors meets a germ with the right antigen, they will fit together perfectly, like a key in a lock.

When a macrophage, coated with particles of partially digested germs arrives in a lymph node, it's like waving a red flag in front of a bull. The B and T cells that have been circulating through your body until this point, looking for something to get excited about, finally get their chance. The antigen presented by the macrophage will match up with receptors on the surface of one or a very small number of T or B cells.

That's all it takes to set the immune cascade in motion.

When a helper T cell that has a receptor that matches up to the germ particles on the macrophage "sees" that stimulus, it immediately starts cloning itself into millions of identical copies. One T cell alone can get the immune response started, but it takes an army of clones to fight off the invaders. Collectively, the cloned helper T cells take over the immune system response. Because they're all identical, you could think of them as the general directing the overall battle, or the coach directing the game. The helper T cells send out chemical signals to the other immune cells that coordinate and amplify the attack. Some of those signals tell B cells to get to work producing antibodies, proteins that attach to the antigens on the invader and tag it for destruction by macrophages and neutrophils. Other helper T cells stimulate more phagocytes to go to the site of the infection and make them eat even faster. The helper T cells put the macrophages into a state of hyperactivation. They get even bigger and more active, hunting down and eating invaders even faster. A hyperactivated macrophage can get so large that it can actually engulf a single-celled parasitic invader.

Helper T cells also send out signals that tell killer T cells to seek out and destroy infected cells, usually cells that are infected by viruses. Killer T cells kill infected cells by making them commit suicide, which kills the virus as well.

Once helper T cells activate B cells, those cells too will clone themselves into millions of copies and start pouring out antibodies to attack the invader. Your body is building up an "army" to mount an attack on the invader. It's this process of cell proliferation that causes a typical sign of any infection: The lymph nodes that drain that area of your body will swell with multiplying T cells and become tender to the touch. Not to worry! Your immune response is doing its job!

When enough cells have built up, they head out of the lymph nodes to kill off the infection. Once they get to the battlefield, chemical messengers are sent from helper T cells. They help stimulate the other immune system cells to keep proliferating and keep attacking. Once the immune response to a bacterial infection gets started and helper T cells are stimulated, these cells will encourage B cells to produce just the right antibody for maximum invader destruction. The B cell antibodies latch onto their counterpart antigens on the germ and mark it for destruction.

The germ becomes studded all over with antibodies, which clog up its cell wall. Antibodies make the germs so attractive and easy to grab that the macrophages and neutrophils gobble even faster. Some types of antibodies can increase the eating speed of phagocytes (phagocytosis) by up to 4,000 times!

Viruses pose a special problem for your immune system. Phagocytes are very good at gobbling up invaders floating around in your blood and tissues, but they can't recognize, much less attack, invaders such as viruses that get *inside* a cell. To solve this problem, Mother Nature has devised a special mechanism to recognize infected cells and kill them specifically. This stops the virus in its tracks, while sparing uninfected cells.

This special signaling system is called the major histocompatibility complex (MHC). It's a group of signaling molecules worn on the surfaces of all your cells. The MHC molecules are like a team uniform that tells your immune system that "you" are "you." When the cells of your body are operating normally, these molecules express an "I'm OK" signal to your white blood cells. If a virus enters a cell, however, the MHC molecules change their appearance, and the cell stops giving off the "I'm OK" signal. Killer T cells see the altered molecules that are now decorating the surface of the cell and recognize them as distress signals announcing that the cell is infected. When a killer T cell sees the altered signal, it latches onto the infected or damaged cell and delivers a "kiss of death" to it—literally, by injecting chemicals that drill holes in the surface of the target cell.

In all but the most serious or fast-moving infections, your immune system will mount a counterattack that will destroy the invaders. With repeated exposure to germs, your immune system gets better, faster, and more specific at dealing with them. Repeated exposure also gives you a large collection of T and B memory cells that have seen that particular invader before and will rapidly produce precisely the right antibody to kill it.

Building a strong, efficient immune system with a lot of powerful memory cells doesn't happen overnight. The first time your body was attacked by that particular germ, you probably felt sick for a few days while your immune system built up its counterattack. The next time your body is attacked by the same germ, your immune cells will recognize it immediately and churn out exactly the right response to destroy it. It all happens so quickly that you probably won't even notice.

It's a process that begins in infancy and continues throughout your lifetime. Before you're even born, Mother Nature gives you the basic tools to create a strong immune system. The rules I'll give you in the next section will help you use those tools wisely.

# PART TWO

------------------------------

# The 5 Cardinal Rules for a Strong Immune System

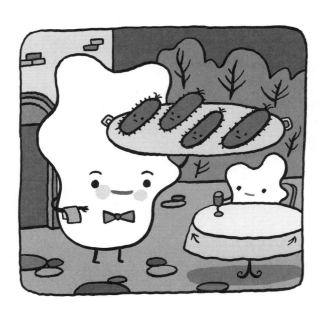

# RULE 1:

# Let Them Eat Dirt: Boot Camp for Young Cells

Kids eat dirt—it's what they do. Young children put absolutely everything in their mouths. First-time parents watch in dismay as their crawling youngsters roll through life like little vacuum cleaners, putting every piece of awful detritus they can find into their mouths with supreme delight. Well, dirt isn't exactly sterile, but it's not necessarily harmful either.

One of my fondest memories of my children is of a day when they were small.

As we built a barn for our horses, my son lay on a blanket in the back pasture, in close range. When I turned around to check on them, I saw my son had crawled over to a dried pile of horse manure and was chewing on it with relish, as if it were a Big Mac. This was the happiest child in the state of Montana. Who are we to try to thwart such a strong biologic urge?

I am certainly not advocating feeding your children a diet of horse manure or other unsavory materials, but I am proposing that we examine why it is that young children are so compelled to put things in their mouths. Certainly, much of it has to do with teething, but the other much more critical role of this behavior is in the training of a young, naïve immune system.

At the teething stage, which normally lasts for the first two years of life, the child's immune system is very immature. The child has just emerged from the sterile environment of the womb and has huge numbers of young, ignorant immune cells circulating through its body. It is the exposure to the less-than-sterile environment of the world that starts these young cells learning their jobs. Like the child itself learning to crawl, then walk, and ultimately run, the early stages of immunological learning are largely by trial and error.

The first natural exposure to the environment occurs during passage through the mother's birth canal. The normal bacterial inhabitants of this area probably provide the child's first dose of the normal flora that will soon colonize her external surfaces and digestive system. Interestingly, children delivered by Caesarian section (and therefore not passing through the birth canal) are more prone to the development of asthma and allergies than are their "naturally" delivered counterparts.

Is it possible that our current obsession with cleanliness is actually counterproductive to health? I am quite certain that it is! But more on that when I get to rule 2.

# Young Immune Cell Training

The processes that protect the human body from infection by viruses, bacteria, fungi, and parasites are extremely complicated cell-to-cell interactions that require practice for perfected execution. Young immune cells released from the bone marrow and thymus have never responded to anything before, so the initial steps of cell-to-cell interaction are a lot like finding a needle in a haystack. Each time a response occurs, the pathways of communication are strengthened, the cells are multiplied, and the size of the immunological army expands.

Naïve cells that have never been exposed to the foreign substance for which they are specifically designed have a very short life span and not much chance to meet up with that substance. But once T cells and B cells have gone through a round of stimulatory signals and become memory cells, they become very long lived and will protect the body for years into the future. Although memory B cells are believed to have a life span of about 10 years, there is evidence that some memory T cells may last most or all of a lifetime. Aged survivors of the great 1918 flu pandemic still had robust antibody production nearly a century later. Clearly, the more exposure to the environment a child has in those early formative years, the more ability he will have to withstand the pathogens of the future.

# Learning How Not to Get Sick

As a fetus develops in its mother's womb, the components of the immune response are already being formed, just as are the heart, lungs, brain, and liver. Inside the uterus the environment is sterile, so virtually no exposure to foreign substances occurs. The exceptions are chemicals that enter the bloodstream. They can be carried across the placenta, so women who abuse drugs and alcohol deliver drug- and alcohol-addicted infants. Some disease agents, such as the virus that causes rubella (German measles) can cross the placenta as well, but these are exceptions to the rule.

Even so, critical steps in the fetus's immunologic education are occurring. The fetal bone marrow and liver are important sources of white blood cells — a fetus is already starting to produce these cells early in gestation. Complex processes in the fetal bone marrow and liver are causing the development of a huge diversity of cells, each with unique receptors for foreign substances, such as the antigens and toxins produced by invading bacteria. Since the child's immune system has no idea what it will meet in its environment after birth, Mother Nature takes the approach of pumping out the maximum possible number of young immune cells with the maximum amount of diversity. By starting life with plenty of immune cells with plenty of diversity, the child is equipped by Mother Nature to handle whatever nasty pathogens Mother Nature later throws at him or her.

The cells that are destined to become T cells are born from stem cells in the bone marrow. From there, they travel to the thymus, a very large organ found in the chest of a child (by adulthood, the thymus has shrunk and is much smaller). The thymus lies over the heart and lungs and is protected inside the rib cage. Mother Nature has designed your body so that all of your most important organs are protected by a bony casing, and the thymus is no exception. That the thymus is so carefully protected in this way confirms current medical thinking that it is the master organ of your immune system.

Once a young T cell arrives in the thymus, its higher education gets started. The young cell develops receptors on its surface that are capable of recognizing proteins (antigens) produced by invaders. Each one of the millions of T cells that pass through your thymus will develop its very own receptor, one that is different from the receptor on any other young T cell. The outside of the T cell will be studded with thousands of its own unique receptors. To make sure each receptor design is a useful one that will be able to respond to an invasion efficiently, T cells need to be trained.

Success here is critical to the ability of your immune system to function properly, so the training a T cell receives in the thymus is extremely rigorous. Somewhere between 90 and 95 percent of the T cells entering the thymus are destined to die there because they fail the "final exam."

That's one tough final. What makes it so hard? The T cell needs to know how to tell the difference between you and an invader — what's known as self/non-self recognition. Within the thymus, a young T cell is shown the molecules that tell it a cell is part of you — it's shown the "you" team uniform. If that T cell likes the uniform so much that it binds strongly to it, it has just flunked the exam. The last thing your immune system needs is a T cell that thinks it should attack your own cells instead of an invader.

The thymus is merciless. A T cell that binds too strongly or too weakly doesn't get to drop the class or switch to a different major — it gets to kill itself.

## When the Immune System Doesn't Work

In rare cases, children are born with an inherited flaw in some part of the immune system. The famous case of the "bubble boy" is a good example. David Vetter's parents had already lost a son to severe combined immunodeficiency (SCID) when he was just six months old. When David was born in 1972, he was quickly diagnosed with the same hereditary problem, although SCID ordinarily arises in only about one of every 100,000 births. David's immune system failed to produce functioning T cells, and his B cells were defective. His body was incapable of mounting an immune response. To keep him from dying of massive infection, David was placed in a sterile incubator, where he was cared for through built-in gloves.

David went from his sterile incubator in the hospital to a sterile plastic "bubble" there, and then eventually to a bubble in the living room of his parent's house. David was allowed no contact with the outside world. His environment was completely germ free: His air was filtered, his food, his clothing, and even his toys were sterilized, and he was able to reach out of his bubble only through built-in gloves. On the rare occasions when he left his bubble, David wore a sort of space suit.

*cont'd on next page*

At first, David's doctors hoped his immune system would eventually mature and start working. By the time David was 12, it was very clear this would never happen and that nothing could ever stimulate his immune system into action. In an effort to give David a normal life, he underwent a bone marrow transplant. The transplant failed and David died in 1984. Later researchers discovered that David's T cells had a defect in the receptor for a communication molecule called interleukin-2, which signals T cells to multiply.

David's case was unusual in the extreme measures used to prolong his life, but in fact primary immunodeficiency diseases—hereditary immune system malfunctions—aren't that uncommon. Researchers have identified more than 70 different types of primary immunodeficiency diseases. Some of these diseases are relatively mild. They can be treated by treating infections as they arise and taking steps to reduce exposure to germs, such as frequent hand washing and avoidance of crowds. More serious cases, such as SCID, can sometimes be markedly improved or even cured by a bone marrow transplant, which gives the child stem cells that will produce working immune system cells to replace his defective ones.

A T cell that passes the final exam is fortunate indeed. Successful T cells clone themselves into millions of identical copies. They then "graduate" and are allowed to leave the thymus and enter your body, where they circulate and linger in your lymph nodes and spleen. As they mature, they will become the helper T cells and killer T cells that will protect you for the rest of your life.

## A Day in the Life of a T Cell

Just like a lot of recent graduates, newly created T cells don't yet have a career path. A young T cell is called immature or naïve, because its receptors haven't yet met up with their counterpart antigens. Until that happens, the young T cell can't do much except hang around, mostly in your lymph nodes and spleen, hoping to meet up with the right antigen that will stimulate it to multiply. If it doesn't find its counterpart antigen within a few days, the young cell will die.

Let's assume that an invader that has just the right antigen on its surface manages to enter your body. Your innate immune system responds immediately by both attacking the invader directly and also sending out help signals to the rest of your immune system.

The request for help reaches your immature T cells by messenger. Macrophages and B cells both attack invaders; when they do, pieces of the invaders end up being displayed on the surface of the immune cells. To get technical about it, immune cells displaying bits of an invader are called antigen presenting cells (APCs).

If the right T cell meets up with an immune cell displaying the right antigen, the T cell's receptors lock on to the antigens, pulling the two cells close together. The end result is that the immature T cell is activated and ready to go to work.

The activated T cell is now presented with a major career choice: It can become a type of helper T cell that will assist in the production of antibodies, or it can become a type of helper T cell that will assist other cells called killer T cells, whose job is to identify cells of your body that are infected with things like viruses. This decision is made in response to what sort of invader the T cell is facing. If the invader is extracellular — that is, it invades your body but stays in the spaces between your cells — then the activated helper T cell will specialize in stimulating and directing your B cells to produce the right antibodies to attack the invader. If the invader is an intracellular one — that is, one that invades the body and lives inside your cells — then the activated helper T cell will stimulate the production of killer T cells, which will hunt down germ-infected cells and kill them before they can spread disease to other cells.

## T Cell Memory

If all goes well, one of the two pathways of T cell activation — antibody helper or helper for killers — will result in the destruction of the invader. When the invader is a bacterium or fungus, the antibody response is most useful. Helper T cells stimulate and direct your B cells to make antibodies against the invader, which in turn lets them be eaten by phagocytes or dissolved by complement. Cell-mediated immunity using killer T cells is most important in cases where your body is attacked by viruses or other intracellular disease-causing agents such as some bacteria, parasites, and fungi.

Once the invader is destroyed, most of the activated T cells will die off. If they didn't, your body would get clogged up with them. Since there was so much cellular multiplication during the activation phase, your population of T cells specific for this particular invader is now much, much larger than it was at first, even though most of the cells have died. The remaining activated T cells live on. They return to their former resting state and become memory cells, hiding out in your lymph nodes and spleen. Because they have already been activated against that particular germ, if it tries to attack you again, your memory T cells snap back into action quickly, and your immune response will be stronger, faster, and more effective.

# Primary and Secondary Immune Responses

When you make an immune response to one germ, the response initially depends on that one specific T cell or B cell, with an appropriate receptor that was created that day. After this cell has become stimulated, the primary immune response happens: It clones itself into zillions of copies, all of which are specific for that same germ. When the infection is cleared, those cells become memory cells, and patrol your body aggressively to prevent this germ from getting in again. If it does, then your immune system will go through a secondary immune response: Another round of activation and cell proliferation will build up into an army yet again. The secondary immune response happens quickly and efficiently—you may not even feel sick while it happens. Your body can make a multitude of these responses every minute of every day.

# Immunity Begins in Infancy

The thymus operates at its peak of activity only during the early years of life. Although experts disagree on the exact timing, it is clear that by the time a child reaches adolescence, the large, robust thymus of early childhood has become a fibrous scar of its former self. What this means to the functioning of the immune system is that there is actually only a fairly small window of opportunity in a human life when T cells can be produced in massive numbers and set loose to patrol your borders. If the final steps of T cell training are not successfully completed during this window of opportunity in the child, it will have lifelong negative consequences for health. Exposure to germs from infancy onward is crucial for developing a lifelong strong immune response.

On the other hand, immunity doesn't happen overnight—the process begins at birth but takes years to develop. What about the germs that attack before the child's immune system is ready to handle them efficiently? As always, Mother Nature has an answer: breastfeeding.

# The Miracle of Maternal Antibodies

One of the small miracles of breastfeeding is the way maternal antibodies are transferred to the infant. When a baby is born, it already has plenty of maternal antibodies circulating in its system. In particular, babies have lots of immunoglobulin G (IgG) antibodies, because these antibodies pass from the mother to the fetus in the womb through the placenta. So, a baby is born with some antibodies to germs that its mother has already been exposed to, which means that the baby is born with some immunity to the germs in the local environment. The maternal IgG antibodies in the baby's body gradually fade away over roughly six months to a year. Not surprisingly, the maternal IgG antibodies wane just as the baby starts making her own IgG.

The chief breastfeeding advantage comes from another maternal antibody called IgA. The first milk to come from a new mother's breast is called colostrum. This thin fluid is crammed with maternal antibodies, especially IgA, that confer passive immunity on the newborn. This is Mother Nature's way of boosting the baby's immune system right at the start with a large dose of maternal antibodies, before the baby's own immune system has matured enough to defend the baby on its own. When the true breast milk starts to appear a day or so later, it is also high in IgA.

The beauty of maternal IgA is that because it passively protects the newborn against infection, it doesn't affect the development of the child's own immune response. The child develops a robust immune response naturally and efficiently, and builds up strong immunity "muscles" at the same time. Even so, children don't usually start making normal adult values of IgA until they're past age two.

Maternal IgA from breast milk isn't actually absorbed into the child's body. Instead, it physically coats the child's vulnerable digestive tract by sticking to the slippery mucosal surfaces. As the child suckles, the IgA antibodies line the mouth, throat, stomach, and intestines. The antibodies form a physical barrier that makes it hard for germs to stick to these areas and attach themselves. They simply pass through the baby and are eliminated along with all the other waste products.

Other substances in breast milk also help provide immune protection for the baby. A protein called lactoferrin, for example, helps prevent bacterial infection by restricting the amount of iron available to bacteria. Without iron, some dangerous bacteria can't take hold and reproduce. One of those bacteria is *Haemophilus influenzae,* the culprit behind many an ear infection or upper respiratory infection in children. Similarly, the enzyme lysozyme keeps some kinds of dangerous bacteria at bay by disrupting the growth of their cell walls. Breast milk is a rich mixture of many other substances as well—substances that we don't begin to understand but that almost certainly play roles in helping infants develop properly and stay healthy.

## Healthier Babies

Breastfeeding has been shown to help prevent many of the common infections babies get. Overall, babies who are entirely or mostly breastfed for at least the first six months don't get as many ear infections, diarrhea attacks, and respiratory tract infections. When they do get sick, they tend to have milder symptoms and get well quicker than bottle-fed babies.

Leaving aside better health for the baby and less wear and tear on the parents, breastfeeding is crucial for helping to reduce the overuse of antibiotics. In general, because breastfed babies don't get sick as much or as severely, they get antibiotics half as often as formula-fed babies. Fewer prescriptions for antibiotics means less chance for developing antibiotic resistance.

Otitis media, well known to all parents as the most common sort of ear infection in young children, is a good example of how antibiotics get overused in kids. Until fairly recently, pediatricians routinely prescribed antibiotics for acute otitis media. American kids get five million cases of acute otitis media each year—75 percent of all kids have had at least one ear infection by the time they reach school age. That many ear infections led to some 10 million prescriptions a year for antibiotics. In fact, half of all the antibiotic prescriptions doctors write for preschoolers are for ear infections. For all the prescriptions, the benefits of antibiotics for treating acute otitis media aren't very great—and about 15 percent of the kids who get them will have diarrhea or vomiting, which could be more harmful than the ear infection itself.

Such heavy prescribing was practically a recipe for creating antibiotic-resistant bacteria, which is indeed what has happened. In 2004 the American Academy of Pediatrics issued new guidelines for treating otitis media. The guidelines call for relieving pain, especially during the first 24 hours, with nonprescription ibuprofen (Advil) or acetaminophen (Tylenol). Antibiotics have no impact on the pain during the first 24 hours and help only slightly after that. For babies who are otherwise healthy and have no underlying conditions, the guidelines call for watchful waiting before prescribing antibiotics. How long to wait? At least 48 hours and as long as 72 hours. About 60 percent of kids will feel much better within two days; after three days 80 to 90 percent feel better. Only those kids who haven't managed to fight off the infection after a few days should get an antibiotic.

The guidelines have definitely reduced antibiotic use for ear infections. Combine the new guidelines with more breastfeeding, and the incidence of ear infections that need antibiotics drops. Studies show that breastfeeding for just three months gives the baby significant protection against ear infections, and that breastfeeding for four or more months reduces the number of ear infections by half. Over the long run, fewer infections to begin with, and milder infections when they do occur, will help lower antibiotic use even more and make a dent in the problem of antibiotic-resistant bacteria.

## Breastfeeding and Allergies

The number of babies and young kids with atopic dermatitis (AD), also known as eczema, has at least doubled in the past three decades. (*Atopic* means a genetic tendency to have an allergic reaction involving IgE antibodies.) Today about 20 percent of kids aged three to 11 have atopic dermatitis. Unfortunately, kids with AD as infants have a strong tendency to develop asthma as they get older—and the number of kids with asthma today is just astounding. The incidence of asthma in young children up to age four increased 160 percent between 1980 and 1994. Today about 54 out of a thousand young kids have asthma, up from about 31 out of a thousand in 1980. The number of kids with allergies to peanuts has doubled in the past decade.

Too much cleanliness probably has a lot to do with pushing the immature immune systems of young children in the direction of allergic responses (I'll go into that more in rule 2). There's another element to the allergy equation, however—breastfeeding. Babies who are breastfed exclusively for at least four to six months are generally much less prone to allergies.

Atopic disease has a strong genetic component—if one or both parents suffer from allergies, their child is very likely to have allergies as well. There's increasing evidence that the genetic tendency toward atopy can be short-circuited by breastfeeding. Studies have shown that in high-risk infants, exclusive breastfeeding for at least four months helps protect against eczema, asthma, and milk allergy in the first two years. This works well for infants who are very likely to develop allergies, based on family history. Exclusive breastfeeding seems to be especially helpful against atopic dermatitis, reducing the incidence in high-risk babies by about a third.

There's no solid evidence that what the mother eats during pregnancy and while breastfeeding has any impact on whether the child will develop food allergies. Having the mother avoid foods that are common allergens, such as peanuts or eggs, doesn't seem to have a preventative effect on food allergies or eczema in the baby. Milk is a substance created in the glandular tissue of the breast. It's made from proteins, fats, and sugars in the mother's body, but eating peanuts doesn't create peanut milk, any more than cows that eat grass make grass milk.

To help prevent allergies in high-risk infants, breastfeeding has to begin at birth. After the infant reaches four to six months, the window for preventing atopic disease through diet seems to close. Switching to breastfeeding or a hypoallergenic formula won't help once the mistaken IgE antibody pathway is established in the immune system.

## The Dirt Factor

One of the most delightful sights for a parent should be a young child covered in dirt from an active afternoon of outdoor play. Unfortunately, that's a sight parents don't see much these days — and when they do see it, they're often horrified. Today too many kids are encouraged to stay indoors, where it's clean and safe and they can't get covered with all those dirty germs. Parents, relax. Kids who play outdoors and get dirty are healthier. They get plenty of physical exercise, and just as important, they get plenty of immunological exercise. Dirt is good for kids.

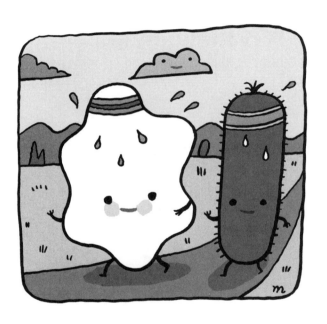

# RULE 2:

# Use It or Lose It: Exercise Your Immune System

Kids who are exposed to plenty of germs from infancy onward develop robust immune systems that will protect them throughout their lives. Their immune systems are "trained" from the very start to recognize the bad guys and react appropriately. If the immune system is pointed in the right direction from the start, the training is more likely to work in desirable ways. There's no substitute for immunologic exercise, starting in infancy, if you want to live a long, healthy life.

White blood cells multiply in response to challenge: Each exposure to a germ gives you more immune cells to respond faster and more aggressively the next time that germ tries to attack. Pretty soon, if that particular germ tries to enter your body, it will be stopped in its tracks so quickly and efficiently that you probably won't even notice. Practice makes perfect, in your immune system as elsewhere. If the white blood cells don't get challenged in early childhood, they don't get any practice in responding correctly. When they are called on to respond, they may not multiply as quickly and correctly as they should for a good immune response. And some types of white blood cells need lots of regular practice. If they don't get it, they start responding in completely wrong ways.

What's the best way to give your immune system the training it needs? Give it dirt.

# The Hygiene Hypothesis

The evidence that a less-than-sterile environment is actually beneficial to young children is common sense that can be demonstrated in a number of different ways. For many years, pediatricians have observed that multiple-child families tend to have better health than single-child families. This is pretty predictable if you follow my "dirt is good for you" hypothesis. Think about the process.

The first-time parents bring their new infant home with all of the best intentions for being the best parents they can possibly be. The home has been child-proofed and they have been carefully coached in the production of a perfectly sterile, safe environment for their little bundle of joy. When that pacifier falls on the floor, the parents cannot throw themselves on it quickly enough to wash it off, soak it in bleach, run it through the dishwasher, the microwave, you name it...anything to make it absolutely sterile before it goes back into that darling little mouth.

Well, Mother Nature has a sense of humor too, so by the time the second child arrives, the blush of new parenthood has been dimmed by several months to years of sleeplessness. When the pacifier is ejected from the mouth of this child, the sleep-deprived mother makes it to the sink, runs it under some water, and plops it back in the child's mouth. By the arrival of the third and subsequent children, parents find pacifiers that have fallen under refrigerators several months before, wipe the dust bunnies off of them, and cram them back into the child's mouth just to stop the screaming.

It's not that you love your second, third, or seventeenth child any less, it's simply that practicality takes control of your life. Fortunately, practicality is Mother Nature's grand design. The child in this family constellation who will have the strongest immune response is the one who saw the most dirt in his early life. The first and most "perfectly" reared child will be the weakest one immunologically.

More formally, "dirt is good for you" is called the hygiene hypothesis. This idea has been around since the 1980s, when doctors and researchers noticed a huge surge in the number of kids being diagnosed with asthma, food allergies, and even type 1 diabetes. At the same time, they noticed a general increase in irritable bowel disease and autoimmune diseases such as multiple sclerosis and rheumatoid arthritis. The hygiene hypothesis ties our modern obsession with cleanliness, along with our increasing tendency to stay indoors in a relatively germ-free and parasite-free environment, to the increase in health problems. When your immune system doesn't get the sort of constant stimulation it has evolved to expect, it doesn't function well. It may get hyperactive and confused. That's when your immune system starts mistaking harmless pollen or food proteins for dangerous invaders, causing allergies, or mistaking your body's own cells for invaders, causing autoimmune diseases.

Of course, allergies and autoimmune diseases existed long before soap was ever invented, but they were rare. Our current allergy and autoimmune epidemics coincide with our new level of cleanliness and excess use of antimicrobials. What we need to reverse the trend is more dirt.

# Learning About Dirt

What a child is doing when he puts things in his mouth is allowing his immune response to explore his environment. Not only does this allow for "practice" of immune responses which will be necessary for protection, but it also plays a critical role in teaching the immature immune response what is best ignored. Learning to distinguish between genuine threats and false alarms is crucial to immune system training. The process begins even before birth.

As discussed in rule 1, a child is protected in the uterus by the immune system of the mother. The placenta, which provides nutrition to the fetus, is like a highly developed pump. It grabs onto maternal antibodies and transports them into the fetal circulation. When the child is born, she already has lots of the mother's antibodies in her circulation. In particular, the child has a lot of immunoglobulin G (IgG for short) antibodies. Your body makes several different classes of antibodies, but only the IgG antibodies pass from the mother to the fetus through the placenta. The IgG antibodies are there to protect infants during the first few months of life, a time when they're not yet able to make them for themselves. Because the mother has already been exposed to the local germs, the IgG antibodies the baby receives will tend to be exactly the antibodies needed to protect her from the germs that are most likely to be in the environment.

After birth, a breastfed baby receives another type of antibody called immunoglobulin A, or IgA for short, from the mother's colostrum and later from her milk. IgA protects the mucous surfaces of the body — including the mouth, throat, and upper digestive tract of the child. In the intestines, the antibodies protect against bacterial infections by coating germs and keeping them from attaching to the intestinal wall. IgA also makes the germs clump together so that they are more easily swept out of the intestines and eliminated in the usual way. Importantly, IgA also protects the entrances from the mouth to the Eustachian tubes leading to the ears. This helps prevent ear infections.

Because maternal IgG and IgA are donated ready-made by the mother instead of being created by the infant, this type of immunity is called passive immunity. The baby doesn't have to do anything to get its protection.

To a newborn child, nutrition is probably the most important stimulus for growth. How does the child's naïve immune system learn the difference between the calories the child requires for life and the invaders which could cause disease? Mother Nature has an answer for this, too.

The presence of maternal IgG and IgA in new babies allows them to concentrate their energy on obtaining calories to grow with. Any pathogen contained in the child's diet will immediately be destroyed by the maternal antibodies, so the child learns to use all his ingested calories for energy—and doesn't learn to make an immune response against his own food. In other words, maternal antibodies help prevent food allergies. How? A baby isn't capable of making IgE antibodies, the ones involved in allergic reactions, until he's well past age two. In the meantime, the baby can make only IgG and IgM antibodies. So, if the baby is going to have any sort of immune response to a food, by definition it will involve only either IgM or IgG antibodies for the first two years. IgM and IgG are helpful antibodies, not allergy causers. Once immune responses using these antibodies are in place, they will get stronger on repeated exposure. The IgE response is the last-ditch effort of the immune system to respond to something that can't be killed in any other way — a parasite, usually. If the baby has plenty of IgG and IgM antibodies, he won't need to make IgE antibodies unless it's absolutely necessary. That means the baby is less likely to develop allergies from mistaken IgE responses.

As the child grows and is continuously exposed to the germs in his environment, his immune system starts to make its own antibodies instead of relying only on passive immunity from the mother. The first antibody class the child will start to make on his own, during the second trimester of gestation, is IgM. The child makes IgM long before his T cells and B cells have figured out how to work together. What makes IgM a great first antibody is that it acts like an immunological sponge. IgM molecules hook themselves together at their tails into groups of five, sort of like a snowflake. By hooking together, they can capture and bind huge amounts of foreign substances very efficiently. The IgM antibodies corral the germs into clumps that are more easily attacked by complement and macrophages and neutrophils.

The infant will start to make his own IgG in response to any foreign substances as soon as he's exposed to the less-than-sterile environment of the world at birth. By the end of the first year of life, the baby is making about 80 percent of the normal adult value of IgG.

It takes quite a bit more time for the child's immune response to learn to make the last two categories of antibodies, IgA and IgE. IgA is the antibody whose role is to protect the mucosal surfaces of the body: your respiratory, digestive, and reproductive tracts. Children don't begin to produce normal adult values of IgA until well into their second year of life. At the end of the first year, the child is only making about 20 percent of normal adult values, and is still susceptible to pathogens that enter the body through the mouth, nose, and other mucosal surface routes.

The antibody molecule that is least likely to be made in these early years of life is IgE, by design. IgE is the antibody of the antiparasite response. It has extremely nasty results, as I'll discuss below, so Mother Nature reserves it for parasites, the most difficult of invaders. This particular antibody will only be made as a last resort, so most children are incapable of making it until past their second year of life.

The IgE molecule is shaped just like IgG, but it has a special tail that allows it to fit into receptors on the surface of mast cells and basophils, the white blood cells that are designed to attack parasites. IgE molecules only exist for a very short period of time when they float free in the bloodstream, but when they become bound to the surface of your mast cells and basophils, they have an extremely long life span.

Antibodies are what make breast milk so important to protect the young child: The mother donates her antibodies, including all the immunoglobulins, and the child is protected passively. This is also the reason why young children are so susceptible to germs that enter the body across these surfaces. In breastfed babies, the IgA they receive may still not be enough to keep germs from entering. Babies that aren't breastfed, of course, don't get any maternal IgA. Passive immunity is imperfect, but that's the idea. Every germ a baby fights and wins against strengthens its immunity for the future.

# Dirt Prevents Allergies

Today we have a lot of very solid evidence showing that early exposure to dirt helps prevent allergies in kids. The cleaner the environment, the more likely a child is to develop allergies; conversely, kids who are exposed to a lot of dirt in early childhood are less likely to develop allergies. To understand why, let's look more closely at the part of your immune system that's involved in allergic reactions. It's the same part that has evolved to protect you from parasites.

Parasites are tiny organisms, such as protozoa and worms, that enter your body and attempt to live there, stealing nutrients from you and causing illness. Obviously this is a bad thing, and your immune system has some robust defenses against parasites. Specifically, your granulocytic white blood cells attack and destroy parasites. Mast cells, basophils, and eosinophils can all dump granules of toxic chemicals on the parasites as a way of forcefully encouraging them to leave your body.

Parasites are a special problem for your immune system. They are the only category of invader in which the foreigner is actually orders of magnitude larger than anything your immune system has to combat it. Parasites such as roundworms, tapeworms, and flukes are extremely complex multicellular creatures, so there's simply no way for any kind of single white blood cell to kill such a huge invader. So what does Mother Nature devise for an invader the relative size of Godzilla? The flamethrower.

If you've ever watched any of the dozen or so versions of the Godzilla story, or if not, the King Kong story, then you have an idea of the relative differences of size between your immune cells (the army) and the invader (Godzilla, King Kong, or the parasite). You probably noticed that bullets, rocket launchers, and so forth did nothing to harm Godzilla. Even so, in the final scenes of the movie she is shown lumbering out into New York harbor, just to get away from the irritation of those puny humans. From the point of view of the average New Yorker, who cares where Godzilla is going as long as she leaves the city? From the point of view of your immune system, convincing worms that your body is not a very nice place to live and that they should go elsewhere would be just fine!

The flamethrowers of your immune system are a group of cells called mast cells, basophils, and eosinophils. The granules inside them contain a nasty concoction of acids that are toxic to everything in their pathway. (If you've ever sprinkled salt on a slug eating the tomatoes in your garden, you have an idea of what happens to the invader.)

Your mast cells hang out just below your mucous surfaces (like in your nose and intestines) and just under the skin. They're on the lookout for invading parasites; the idea is to catch the parasites as soon as they enter your body and before they can penetrate any further. If the mast cells go on the attack against a parasite, they simply explode—they basically napalm the area. Basophils and eosinophils, the other granulocytic parasite-attacking cells, join in. No matter which granulocytic cell is involved, the basic method of attack is the same: Get out the flamethrower.

When worms attempt to get through your skin or mucous membranes, these cells will dump their contents at those sites of penetration, killing the parasite directly or at least encouraging it to move elsewhere. The problem with this particular mechanism is that it's not very precise. Remember what New York City looked like at the end of the Godzilla movie? There were lots of skyscrapers that needed screen doors on their top floors. Likewise, wherever your mast cells and basophils disgorge their toxic contents, many cells die—both your own and those of the invader.

The IgE type of antibodies bind to the surfaces of the granulocytes and serve as a "targeting" device, "aiming" the direction of the flamethrower. It's better than nothing, but IgE antibody targeting isn't a very precise mechanism and it can't prevent the granulocytes from causing lots of damage to your own tissues.

Most parasites get into your body either when you accidentally eat them or their eggs or when immature worms called larvae penetrate the skin. Mother Nature is willing to compromise and let a few worms live in your body, but beyond that, she's going to activate her flamethrower.

If new larvae attempt to penetrate your skin or migrate through your body, IgE antibodies made during the earlier worm attacks will bind to mast cells in the skin and mucosa, and target the worms for destruction. Once the IgE antibodies are cross-linked to the surface of the new invaders — in other words, once the IgE has aimed the flamethrower — the mast cells dump their toxic chemicals onto them. This stops their further development and kills them before they can progress any farther.

# The Backup Flamethrower

Your immune system has a backup system for dealing with parasites. It's called antibody-dependent cell-mediated cytotoxicity. The antibody-dependent part of this approach means that all that's required to activate it is a receptor on the white blood cell (that's the cell-mediated part) that is capable of binding to the tail of an IgG antibody. In other words, the system doesn't need helper T cells to direct it. If the other end of the antibody then attaches to an injured cell or a parasite, toxic chemicals (the cytotoxicity part) are released, which cause the death of the target.

## Allergies

Allergies are an example of a good immune response gone bad. As we have seen, when parasites invade your body, it is difficult to destroy them without also causing some innocent bystander damage. In settings where parasitic disease is common, this is an acceptable compromise. Some worms are allowed to survive and complete their life cycles, while the immune response prevents massive parasite infections that might jeopardize the life of the human host. The parasites themselves do some damage by stealing nutrients from the person, but this isn't generally too much of a problem, at least when the parasite load is relatively low.

There are, of course, a multitude of parasites, such as the one that causes malaria and the blood fluke that causes schistosomiasis, that can evade your immune system and cause serious disease and even death. And even a parasite that a healthy person can usually keep at acceptable levels can multiply rapidly and cause severe illness or even death in very young children, the elderly, and anyone with a compromised immune system, such as someone with AIDS or malnutrition.

In developed countries parasitic diseases are no longer common. Simple precautions, such as wearing shoes to avoid skin penetration and proper sewage disposal to avoid fecal contamination of water supplies, have resulted in a dramatic decline of parasitic disease. Overall, this is a good thing. Parasite infestations can cause serious illness, disability, and even death.

The lack of even a few parasites in your body, however, can be a problem. Some humans are unusually good at mounting the antiparasite response. Unfortunately for them, when there aren't any parasites to respond to, their robust antiparasite talents aren't put to their proper use. In the absence of parasites, their antiparasite response can become misdirected against harmless substances in the normal environment. And when your body unleashes an antiparasite response against something harmless, the damage to your own tissues causes the miserable symptoms of allergies: runny nose, sneezing, hives, diarrhea, and possibly even death by anaphylactic shock.

The allergic response develops in the following way:

1.  The immune system is exposed to an allergen. Any sort of antigen can be allergen — the proteins on the surface of pollen, animal dander, cockroach saliva, some foods such as peanuts and eggs, the chemicals in insect stings, and many other substances are common allergens. Most people have immune systems that can tell the difference between a harmless bit of ragweed pollen and a serious parasitic invader. Some people, though, have immune systems that can't. They see these harmless substances as invaders.

2.  The first exposure to the allergen sensitizes the immune system. Your body produces IgE antibodies against the allergen. That's because the confused immune system thinks the allergen is

a parasite, and IgE antibodies are particularly effective against parasites.

3.  The IgE antibodies attach themselves by their tails to receptors on the mast cells, thinking they are lying in wait for that pesky parasite should it try to return.

4.  What returns instead is the harmless allergen. When the allergen crosslinks the antibodies on the mast cell a reaction is triggered. The mast cell activates its flamethrower (degranulates). Toxic chemicals, including one called histamine, spill out. If there happened to be a parasite nearby, it would be slaughtered. Unfortunately for the allergic person, there aren't any worms, just innocent pollen or cat dander.

5.  When the mast cell chemicals are released, they do all sorts of nasty things to the area around them. Histamine makes nearby blood vessels get leaky, and fluid escapes from them into your tissues, giving you a runny nose, watery eyes, and sneezing. Histamine is also responsible for making the bronchial

tubes in your lungs constrict and fill up with mucus, giving you an asthma attack. If the mast cells lining your digestive tract are activated by a food allergy, the usual result is vomiting or diarrhea. No matter where the mast cells are, the chemicals released by degranulation cause inflammation and tissue damage.

6. When mast cells and basophils degranulate, they produce chemical signals of an allergic reaction. This stimulates your immune system to call out another type of granulocytic cell, the eosinophil. These cells take a little longer to mobilize for action than the quick response of mast cells and basophils. Eosinophils are very important in the tissue remodeling and repair that needs to follow the damage caused by the flamethrowers. They produce a large number of enzymes that neutralize the damage and start the tissue repair process, which is desirable. Unfortunately, repair means scar formation, so tissue that is chronically damaged by allergic

hypersensitivity becomes a fibrous scar that no longer has the same function.

Once the IgE/allergen pathway is "learned" by your immune system, each exposure to the allergen perfects its expression — you become even more reactive to the allergen. Just as the size of your immunologic army is increased beneficially to protect you from harm when there's a real invader, when it's erroneously activated, it still increases in size and causes more and more bystander damage. The only answer to the problem of allergies, once they begin, is avoidance of the allergen until the memory cells of your body have died of old age. The life span of a B lymphocyte memory cell is about 10 years; that of T helper memory cells is probably much longer. Waiting for their death is obviously impractical: It makes much more sense to try to avoid their sensitization in the first place!

# Avoiding Allergies

There's no good reason to have allergies. They don't protect you against anything—all they do is make you miserable. So why do some people have them? To a degree, because they have inherited a tendency toward allergies. To a much larger degree, because they weren't exposed to enough dirt when they were young.

When a naïve T cell gets activated and goes down the helper T career path, it makes a further career choice, becoming a Th1 or Th2 cell. The difference between them is in the types of cytokines they produce—the different chemicals send different messages to the rest of the immune system. All antibodies except IgM are under the control of the Th2 cells.

Kids who get the usual number of childhood infections and are exposed to normal amounts of germs from the dirt around them are less likely to get asthma, because their immune system is tilted away from the IgE pathway. Recent studies have shown that young children who go to day care starting at an early age — between six months and a year old — have a 75 percent lower risk of developing wheezing, which is often an early symptom of asthma, than young children who stay at home. When kids start day care after their first birthday, they have a 35 percent lower risk of wheezing, which shows that the real protection comes during that six-month window of a child's immune development. Kids who live in extra clean environments, don't go to day care in early childhood, and aren't allowed to play outside and get dirty tend to get allergies because their immune systems aren't challenged enough. Without those challenges, their immune systems can tilt toward the IgE pathway.

If the immune response in a child is allowed to develop normally, with normal "dirt" in the environment, then IgE should be the very last thing that would be produced. Any germ that required an immune response should first cause production of IgM, the most common type of antibody, followed by IgG and then IgA, depending on how the germ managed to enter your body. As long as these protective responses are strong and successfully remove the pathogen, there will be no further stimulus to make IgE antibodies.

It used to be medical dogma that children from "atopic" families (those with an inherited tendency to allergies) should be protected from early exposure to things against which they might develop allergies. Current medical thinking is exactly the opposite. Those small, random exposures to harmless things in the environment "train" the immune response to function to the benefit of the child, not its detriment. It stands to reason that if you shield the child from normal exposures until he's capable of making IgE after the age of two, you are simply predisposing the perfection of the IgE response and predisposing the child to the formation of IgE against harmless substances. Put more simply, *too little dirt predisposes to allergies.*

Once again, the medical literature supports the common sense. Children raised in rural and farm environments have fewer allergies, even though their exposures to pollen, animal fur, and so on are greater than those of children raised in urban environments. Up until recently, the response of a family suffering lots of allergies was to try to raise their children in an environment free of those allergens so that they would not develop the problems of the parents. Unfortunately, this just makes the problem multigenerational. Children raised in "overclean" environments don't develop normal immune responses. They suffer the double jeopardy of too little protection from harmful germs and too much response to harmless things.

Once the pathway to make IgE instead of less damaging antibodies is established, it becomes a more and more likely response to the environment. Individuals who become good at making this antibody are actually at a strong selective advantage in environments where parasites are common. In our parasite-free society, however, that advantage becomes a disadvantage. These individuals suffer from the flamethrower aspects of the immune response.

Once the immune response has been trained in the allergic direction, it is extremely difficult to "reprogram" it. These individuals tend to become more and more allergic over their lifetimes. The only hope in these cases is to stop the development of this response before it becomes well established.

There's some exciting research in this direction. One recent approach is to try to prevent the development of allergies in young children who come from families with a strong tendency toward severe allergies. The researchers deliberately infect these kids with parasites. The logic is that the parasites will give the kids' hyperactive immune systems something real to react to and keep them from developing allergies. By using a type of worm that commonly infects pigs but that can't complete its life cycle in humans, the experiment is safe — the worms can't become established and start being harmful. This may sound no more attractive to you than my young son's palate for horse manure, but it makes perfect sense in the context of the design of the immune system. When young children from extremely allergic families (presumably genetically predisposed to make the anti-Godzilla response) are deliberately infected with these worms, it sets the immune response down the right track of mounting an IgE response against a parasite, not an allergen. Then, when the parasite is successfully killed in the tissues, the immune response is correctly programmed to put away the flamethrower and reserve this pathway only for occasions of parasitic infection. These children develop dramatically reduced rates of allergic disease compared to their parents.

## Autoimmune Diseases

Mothers through the ages have tormented their children with the adage, "The idle mind is the devil's playground!" This is because mothers instinctively know that if you are not doing your homework, mowing the lawn, cleaning the house, or doing a list of assigned chores, you will surely be out at the mall smoking dope. Your immune response is no different. If it is occupied with protecting you from a dirty environment, it has no time to be out looking for trouble. If it has nothing better to do because its environment is superclean, then it can cause the damage of allergy and autoimmunity.

Autoimmune diseases are those in which your immune response either fails to learn correctly, or forgets its training of what "you" look like. The incidence of autoimmune diseases tends to increase as we age, probably because the decreasing function of the thymus over time makes it harder for your immune system to tell self and nonself apart. The immune response depends on the "command" of its "generals," the T helper cells. When these decline in number with age, the cells that depend on your T helper cells for direction may receive inappropriate signals and begin to mount immune responses against your own tissues.

Autoimmune diseases are some of the most difficult diseases that medicine faces today. They include type 1 (childhood) diabetes, lupus erythematosus, multiple sclerosis, rheumatoid arthritis, and many others. When the immune system learns self/nonself recognition incorrectly, the entire system eventually conspires to rid itself of the perceived invader. If that "invader" is you, then it is easy to see that the outcome will not be positive. The only solution to these diseases is the broad-spectrum immunosuppression of the patient through drugs that kill or inhibit the action of T cells. This by definition inhibits the entire immune response (both good and bad) and the patient becomes susceptible to all the minor germs in the environment.

There is increasing evidence that normal, everyday infections in our youth may prevent the onset of autoimmune disease. Since 1960, we have seen a tripling of the number of cases of type 1 diabetes in children under 15 in the United States and Europe. In a mouse model for diabetes, multiple minor infections in young animals appeared to prevent its onset.

## System Failure: HIV, T Cells, and AIDS

Unfortunately for humankind, the human immunodeficiency virus (HIV) is truly the perfect immunological pathogen.

HIV infects and kills all of your helper T lymphocytes and all of your macrophages. As the disease progresses, all the immune responses that are under the control of helper T lymphocytes cease to function. Since every immune defense you have depends on regulation by these cells, once they decline below a critical level the body is hopelessly susceptible to every single substance in the environment, including opportunistic infections — infections caused by pathogens that don't usually cause illness in people with a healthy immune system. At this point the patient has progressed to acquired immunodeficiency syndrome, better known as AIDS.

## The Immune Response During HIV Infection

Early in the infection, your body responds to HIV just as it would for any other viral infection. But just as the immune response against it begins, the virus goes into hiding inside the chromosomes of the infected cells. Because the very cells that should be protecting you against infection are themselves infected, HIV now has the perfect way to reproduce. When someone with HIV has an immune response, even to the most ordinary, everyday germs, the virus replicates right along with the proliferating T cells. Why? Because the first thing any self-respecting lymphocyte does in response to infection signals is to clone itself, which is exactly what the infected helper T cells do when they detect an infection. When HIV-infected T cells clone themselves, the virus gets cloned, too. That increases the amount of the virus in the body (the viral load). The greater your viral load, the faster your progression to AIDS.

Because the HIV-infected cells are helper T cells and macrophages, as the virus kills them off, or as your own immune response kills them, eventually your number of helper T cells decreases to a dangerously low level. You no longer have enough T cells to recognize invading pathogens and send signals to activate the rest of the immune system, and you can no longer mount an immune response to anything. Harmless pathogens that ordinarily would be easily dealt with by someone with a normal immune response can fatally infect someone with AIDS.

## The Dirt Factor

That old saying, "What doesn't kill you makes you stronger," definitely applies to your immune system. I'm not suggesting life-threatening infections are a good thing—they're not—but your immune system only gets stronger from being attacked. From infancy onward, every germ you fight off increases your ability to fight that germ off again later on even more effectively. Every germ you fight off also strengthens the communications among your immune system cells and lets you mount an offense against an invader that much more quickly. When your immune system doesn't encounter a lot of dirt, it doesn't get challenged. Instead of responding quickly and accurately to germs, it reacts slowly, leaving you open to more frequent and severe illness. And when kids don't get exposed to enough dirt, their immune systems start making the sort of serious mistakes that can lead to autoimmune illnesses, allergies, and asthma. When your immune system is exposed to plenty of dirt on a regular basis starting when you're very young, it gets the regular workouts it needs to build up defenses and stay ready for action.

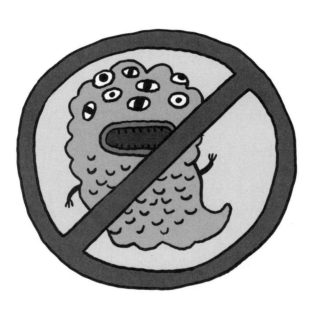

## RULE 3:

# Don't Encourage Superbugs: Avoid Antimicrobics Whenever Possible

I can hear all those germophobe Matt Lauers and Adrian Monks protesting that "it's a jungle out there" and that it's an absolute necessity to protect yourself from getting sick by carrying hand sanitizers and wipes and sporting a face mask. Not so. The only true defense against illness is a strong, healthy immune response and the only way to accomplish that is through repetitive exposure.

When we surround germs with an environment that is constantly full of disinfectants, antimicrobial soaps, and antibiotic drugs, they quickly evolve to resist these chemicals. Germs are living creatures — they adapt to their environment just as we do. The difference is that while humans create a new generation in the United States on average every 27 years, bacteria and many other pathogens can produce new generations literally in minutes. They can far outdistance us in their ability to adapt quickly to their environment.

One result of our societal trend toward germophobia, supercleanliness, and heavy antibiotic use is weakened individual immunity due to lack of dirt. That's bad enough, but we've also created evolutionary selection for the production of new "superbugs" — pathogens that can't be killed by the usual sanitation methods and that resist antibiotic drugs. The age of antibiotics — the miracle drugs such as penicillin that have saved countless lives — is perilously close to coming to an end. The blame lies squarely with us.

# Treating Infections

Antimicrobial agents are drugs that selectively target the germs that enter our bodies. They can be classified as antibacterials, antivirals, antifungals, or antiparasitics. The word *antibiotic* is usually reserved for the natural products of some organisms that inhibit the growth of others (penicillin, for example, which is produced by a mold). More broadly, the word is often used to mean any drug that targets agents of infectious disease.

Because each category of invading agent has a unique anatomy and life cycle, the drugs we use to combat them must be specifically targeted toward them. For example, many antibacterials such as tetracycline target a unique molecule in the bacterial cell wall; the drug makes the cells explode. Because human cells don't have cell walls, these drugs don't harm the human host. Similarly, many antifungals target a unique molecule in the cellular membrane of those life-forms, and therefore have a selective toxicity only for fungi.

Viruses are parasitic on our cells. They hijack them to complete their life cycle, so it's difficult to develop drugs that work against viruses without also harming the human cells in which they live. Antibacterials don't slow the virus life cycle in any way, so there's no point in taking these medications when the agent infecting you is a virus, not a bacterium.

There are only a few antiviral drugs on the market today, which is actually fortunate, because we are still forced to use our own immune systems to defend ourselves against viruses. Drug resistance in these groups is thus much less common than it is among the bacteria.

Parasites have cells that are quite similar to our own, which means that finding unique target molecules for antiparasitics can be difficult. Again, antibacterials, antivirals, and antifungals typically only work on one group of organisms and will not work on parasites.

Our desire to overwash, overbathe, and overmedicate our bodies causes changes in the normal populations of organisms (flora) that live in and on us. Normal flora aren't just harmless hitchhikers on your body. You actually need them, because they're necessary for protecting you from infection from more harmful bacteria. Normal flora fill up all the sites in and on our bodies — living on our skin, our hair, our mucous membranes. Dangerous bacteria have to compete hard for a space on your body. Because they're way outnumbered by harmless and good bacteria, bad bacteria have a hard time getting a foothold, much less finding a space with exactly the right environment for them to grow. For example, normal flora maintain the normal acid/base balance of any place where they live, including you. Pathogens like their environment a little more acidic or basic than the normal flora do. If you have a good balance of normal flora, pathogens won't be able to find a good place to live on you.

When you need to clean your hands, your body, or your house, simple soap and water will do the job. Get rid of all those antimicrobial soaps, germ-killing antiseptic sprays, hand wipes, kitchen and bath sanitizers. All you are doing by using them is killing the harmless and helpful normal flora of your body and helping the harmful organisms around you develop resistance to the very chemicals you are using to try to kill them.

When we overclean our bodies and our environments, the populations of normal flora get disrupted—and pathogenic organisms take advantage of the change in environment and lack of competition to grow. When we constantly medicate minor infections with antimicrobics, it causes the normal flora to adapt by developing mutations that protect them from a chemical-laden environment. And once normal flora organisms adapt to this new environment and develop resistance to all the chemicals surrounding them, they can transfer their resistance to other, more dangerous germs. That this will happen isn't just possible, it's certain.

In fact, antibiotic resistance began almost as soon as there were antibiotics. Penicillin became widely available to the public in 1944, and by 1947, doctors were reporting cases of resistant *Staphylococcus aureus,* the bacterium responsible for many skin infections and also deadly toxic shock syndrome. To kill off this bacterium, doctors switched to methicillin. By 1961, methicillin-resistant *Staphylococcus aureus* (MRSA) had developed, and by the 1980s it was widespread in hospitals. Today, about three-quarters of all *S. aureus* infections in the United States are MRSA. Most occur in hospitalized patients who are already very ill. Community-acquired MRSA, however, is now a worrisome and growing problem. These infections occur among the general population of people living in the community. MRSA passes among community members by skin-to-skin contact with an infected person, by contact with shared personal items such as razors and towels, by crowded living conditions, and by poor hygiene.

By the late 1990s, vancomycin, the only drug left for treating MRSA, had stopped working. Vancomycin-resistant *Staphylococcus aureus*, or VRSA, is now well established in hospitals around the world. Many other harmful bacteria, such as *Enterococcus faecium,* which causes severe diarrhea, and *Streptococcus pneumoniae,* which causes pneumonia, have also developed drug resistance.

# What's Wrong with Antibacterial Soap

With all those superbugs out there, the natural germophobe reaction is keep yourself and your environment even cleaner using even stronger antiseptics. After all, you can die from one of those horrible infections, right? That's exactly the wrong approach—in fact, it's the approach that might actually make you more, not less, vulnerable to infection. Your own immune system and plain old soap and water will keep you healthy.

Ordinary soap and water work just fine for washing your hands (and the rest of you). What you're doing when you use soap to wash is physically removing dirt and its accompanying germs from your skin. The foaming action of the soap helps the process along by dissolving grease and skin oils, but basically, you're simply using friction to rinse the germs away. You're not trying to kill them and sterilize your skin — you're just trying to temporarily wash them off. Plain soap and water clean very effectively.

What happens when you add an antibacterial drug such as triclosan to your soap? You already know: You kill off all the susceptible germs and give the resistant germs an edge by eliminating their competition. In addition, the lingering effects of the drug make it harder for good bacteria to recolonize your skin after you wash. What's the result of that? More opportunities for bad bacteria to colonize you instead.

The primary ingredient in the hundreds of liquid antibacterial soaps on the market today is triclosan. In much higher concentrations, triclosan is used in hospital settings — by surgeons scrubbing before an operation, for example. At those concentrations and in that setting, triclosan kills bacteria across the board. At the much lower concentrations in soap made for consumer use (usually 0.15 percent), the amount of triclosan is just right for creating resistance to it. The same mechanisms bacteria evolve to resist triclosan in soap, such as developing efflux pumps that basically spit drugs out, are exactly the same mechanisms they develop when they become resistant to other antibacterial drugs. The risk that triclosan will drive the development of cross-resistance to other antibacterials is high. The risk is similar for triclocarbon, the antibacterial drug used in bar soaps.

Even worse, while these products are contributing every day to the crisis of antibiotic resistance, there's no evidence that they're actually effective in the sense of providing any health benefit. Antibacterial soaps kill bacteria in the laboratory, but there's very little evidence that they do so in everyday settings.

And on top of that, by using antibacterial soaps on kids—and even giving them toys impregnated with triclosan—we're keeping them from developing and maintaining normal skin and internal flora. The lack of those crucial germs as a child's immune system matures can only contribute to the development of allergies and asthma.

You might be wondering why antibacterial soaps don't have any proven health benefit. Surely having cleaner hands leads to less illness. Actually, that's true, but the fallacy here is that most common illnesses aren't caused by bacteria—they're caused by viruses. Antibacterial soaps have no additional effect whatsoever on the viruses that cause colds, flu, and many intestinal upsets. In fact, numerous studies show that there's no difference in illness rates among people who use antibacterial soaps and those who use plain soap. There is a financial difference, however—antibacterial soaps cost more.

What about the bacteria that cause food-borne illness, such as *Salmonella*? Again, plain soap and water are just fine for hand washing and cleaning kitchen equipment and surfaces. Most of the harmful bacteria will be on and in the contaminated food itself, so a far better approach is prevention by practicing safe food handling and storage and cooking foods thoroughly.

# When Do You Need an Antibiotic?

By killing off good and bad germs indiscriminately, antimicrobics create selection pressure. The germs inevitably adapt to the antimicrobial substances by developing resistance, which means the antimicrobials won't work against them anymore.

My philosophy about antibiotic therapy is that it should be avoided unless your condition is life threatening. This may sound extreme, but remember, every time your body mounts an immune response, it develops immunological memory and gets stronger. Every time you use a quick chemical fix on an illness, you help the germ get stronger but only weaken your immune system.

Needless to say, your physician gets the last word about when you need a prescription. If your doctor says you need to take an antibiotic, do so—and follow the instructions precisely and take the entire prescribed course. When you first start taking an antibiotic, the first germs to die will be the ones that are still sensitive to the drug; the ones that are more resistant will hold out longer. If you stop taking the antibiotic as soon as you feel better (usually in a few days), you are simply compounding the problem of drug-resistant organisms. An experiment in evolution is happening right in your body—you're naturally selecting for those organisms resistant to low levels of the drug. As soon as you stop taking the drug, the resistant organisms will begin to multiply wildly. The next time you need that drug, it will no longer be effective. By taking every pill in the prescription bottle exactly as directed, you stand a good chance of killing off even the resistant organisms.

Good communication with your physician is paramount. Many doctors simply prescribe antibiotics because it is the easy and expected thing to do, or because they feel pressured by the patient to prescribe something. If you tell your doctor that you would prefer a conservative approach to medications, she will be happy to honor your wishes. If you've established this with your doctors, when they do feel medication is strongly advisable, you'll know that it really is.

Today most physicians understand that handing out antibiotics for every little infection, even if they're not sure it's caused by a bacterium, isn't a good idea. Automatically prescribing antibiotics for ear infections and sinusitis, for example, is now frowned on by medical guidelines. Of course, to the uncomfortable patient (or the parent of the screaming baby), a magic pill to "cure" the infection is just what they want. They will often insist on antibiotics. Chances are, however, that the infection is caused by a virus, in which case the antibiotic is useless. Antibiotics can be lifesavers in serious bacterial illness such as meningitis and pneumonia—and they should be reserved for such cases.

Your immune system will clear up most minor bacterial illnesses within a week. Taking an antibiotic may speed up the process by a couple of days, but antibiotics have a down side for the patient. Allergic reactions, skin rashes, digestive upsets, diarrhea from killing off beneficial bacteria in the intestines, and even liver and kidney damage can happen. In fact, bad reactions to antibiotics cause an estimated 142,000 visits to the emergency room every year. Whenever possible, let your immune system do what it's designed to do rather than relying on antibiotics. You'll be building your immunological strength while helping to slow the spread of antibiotic resistance.

# The Problem of Antibiotic Resistance

Antibacterials in the penicillin family of drugs act by inhibiting the formation of the cell wall of bacteria. They bind to proteins found in the cell membrane of the bacterium and fatally weaken the rigid structure of the cell wall. In the 1980s we began to see methicillin-resistant *Staphylococcus aureus* (MRSA), which had developed a mutation in one of those proteins and therefore had become resistant to penicillin and methicillin. *S. aureus* infections are common among seriously ill patients in hospitals. In 1974, the percentage of patients in hospital intensive care units with resistant *S. aureus* infections as compared to nonresistant *S. aureus* was 2 percent. By 1995, that figure had risen to 22 percent; by 2004, MRSA amounted to 64 percent of all *S. aureus* infections. By 1997, we had begun to see vancomycin resistance in another type of bacterium, *Enterococcus*, and by 2002, *Enterococcus* had donated the vancomycin resistance gene to MRSA, creating vancomycin-resistant *Staphylococcus aureus* (VRSA). This is an extremely frightening development because VRSA is an organism against which we truly have no medical means of control.

MRSA has high costs — and they're getting higher. According to the federal Centers for Disease Control (CDC), which is in charge of tracking infectious diseases, between 1999 and 2005, the estimated number of MRSA-related hospitalizations more than doubled, from 127,036 to 278,203. Of those patients, a significant percentage died from their infection — in 2005, nearly 7,000 Americans died of MRSA-related causes.

The annual cost to treat people with MRSA runs to many millions of dollars.

# Wash Your Hands

For most health problems, prevention is far easier than treatment. Hospitals today are working hard to prevent MRSA and VRSA infections by improving standard procedures to reduce the risk of infection and taking strong steps to keep the infection from being passed on to other patients. At the top of the list for prevention is hand sanitation — wearing gloves, washing hands often, and using alcohol-based hand sanitizers when hand washing is inconvenient.

I'm not advocating hospital-level cleanliness in daily life. I'm certainly not advocating the constant use of antimicrobial hand wipes or gels or washing your hands with antimicrobial soap every time you touch something that has germs on it. Everything you touch all the time has germs on it, and trying to sterilize yourself is futile. All you have to do to stay healthy is wash your hands with plain old soap and water as needed.

The reason hand washing with plain soap and water helps cut back on your risk of catching something is simply because you're rinsing away bacteria and viruses. That cuts down on the chances that you'll touch your mouth, nose, face, or some other orifice and introduce the germ into your body. Washing your hands also reduces the risk of transmitting germs to someone else. This is extremely important in health-care settings and when you're in contact with infants and people with weakened immunity from chronic illness, chemotherapy, or some other health problem.

Hand washing can help cut down a bit on the number of colds and minor illnesses you get over the course of a year. It's also very helpful for cutting back on food-borne illnesses. According to the Centers for Disease Control, poor hand washing, or not washing at all, accounts for nearly half of food-borne illness outbreaks. Millions of people get sick each year from food-borne illnesses, and about 5,000 people a year in the United States die from food-borne illnesses such as salmonellosis or infection with *Campylobacter* or *Escherichia coli*.

Because I don't advocate getting sick any more than you have to, or passing illnesses on to others, I certainly recommend washing your hands after using the bathroom, before eating, after changing a diaper, before and after handling food, whenever they're visibly soiled, and so on. That's just common sense. In addition, the diminished population size of germs that will remain on your skin after simple washing will provide a constant stimulus for your immune response to flex its muscles and remain strong.

The average person washes his hands for just five seconds, which doesn't do much to rinse away germs. For maximum effectiveness, hand washing with plain soap and water should last for 20 seconds; any longer doesn't really remove any more germs.

## Hand Sanitizers

Plain alcohol-based hand sanitizers are useful when there's no running water nearby and you absolutely must clean your hands. The alcohol kills germs across the board and doesn't seem to create antibiotic resistance. Avoid hand sanitizers that also contain an antimicrobial ingredient—you're just adding to the problem when you use them. Ditto for hand wipes and household wipes that contain antibiotics. Hospital studies have shown that antibacterial alcohol wipes don't so much kill germs as just spread them around—the wipes have been shown to transfer drug-resistant bacteria from one surface to another rather than killing them.

If you must use a hand wipe, choose the kind meant for babies, which don't contain antimicrobials or alcohol. For household cleaning, wipes may be convenient, but they're not really sanitizing any better than plain soap and water. They also contain chemicals that are harmful to the environment. If you must use these products, choose a brand without an antimicrobial.

You don't really need all those antimicrobial disinfectants for cleaning the house, either. Today there are many "green" cleaning products that contain only simple, environmentally safe ingredients such as pure liquid soap, distilled white vinegar, and baking soda. These products clean perfectly well but don't contribute to drug-resistant bacteria. They don't contain harmful chemicals that you probably shouldn't breathe in, and they don't damage the environment.

## Bacterial Sex: How Bacteria Become Drug Resistant

Every time you use an antimicrobial product, even for the best of reasons such as preventing infection in a hospital, you're contributing to the problem of drug resistance. You might not think that your actions, taken on something way too small to see, could have much of an impact, but they do. Bacteria reproduce very rapidly, and they evolve extremely rapidly to adapt to their environment. You can kill some of them, but the ones that are left will be those that have adapted to resist your efforts. They're the ones that will reproduce.

Bacteria divide by binary fission—an asexual process that involves division of one bacterium into two, two into four, and so on. Because binary fission is asexual, the only way to create new genetic variants is by mutation (new variation can't come from the random mixture of genes from two parents, as in sexual reproduction). A mutation is an accidental error in the DNA coding of an organism. Most mutations are harmful and the organism dies before it can pass the mutated genetic code on, but every now and then a mutation will, just by chance, be good for the organism. A bacterium with a useful mutation—a thicker cell wall that is more resistant to penicillin, for instance—will out-reproduce others that don't have the mutation, and the gene for the mutation will become more prevalent in the population.

Bacteria have developed rapid and efficient means of trading genes, including resistance genes, with one another. This means that future generations of these bacteria will have increased proportions of those resistant forms. The more we use antibacterials, the worse the problem becomes.

Living beings compete with others in their environments for food, shelter, and other resources. If food is scarce, for example, then an individual capable of being more energy efficient and surviving on less food is at an advantage and might be the only member of his species able to reproduce himself. If others die of starvation or are unable to reproduce, then their genes are lost to the population, and the genes of the stronger individual will become a larger proportion of the total gene pool for that species. Evolution is the way that Mother Nature makes certain that the strong survive. The process applies to all of her creations: viruses, bacteria, fungi, parasites, and *us*!

If you think about this process as it pertains to the germs that infect us, you realize that we are providing exactly the right sort of selection pressure to ensure that disease agents become more and more difficult to kill. When there are 100 germs in a location and you kill 99 of them, then the one bacterium whose genes make it more resistant to whatever you used to kill the other germs (in other words, the one capable of surviving the death blow) is the one that will survive and go on to reproduce many more of its kind. Now you have accidentally pushed evolution in the direction of selecting for this mutant strain. The next time you try to use this particular method or drug to destroy that germ, it won't work on the new, tougher organism.

The genes that encode bacterial drug resistance may be found on the bacterial chromosome, on plasmids (tiny circles of DNA) inside the cell, or even in the DNA of viruses that live inside bacteria (bacteriophages). The chromosome of a bacterium is a large, closed circle of DNA that floats in the cell. (Bacteria are prokaryotic, which means they don't have a nucleus to enclose their DNA. A bacterium's single chromosome contains about 2,000 genes; by contrast, humans have 23 chromosomes and about 30,000 genes). If even one of these genes mutated, it would probably cause the death of the organism, because mutations are almost always harmful. Every now and then, however, a mutation turns out to be beneficial—and it was a mutational change that resulted in the development of one of the nastiest germs in our present day environment, methicillin-resistant *Staphylococcus aureus* (MRSA).

Many of the genetic changes that make a bacterium resistant to antibiotics don't occur in the chromosome. They happen in the plasmids, where a harmful mutation is less likely to kill the bacterium. And because bacteria can readily transfer plasmids among themselves, a fortunate plasmid mutation can spread very rapidly.

Bacteria have three basic "strategies" for resisting the actions of our drugs. They're not deliberate actions on the part of the bacteria. Evolutionary pressures have selected for the strategies—those bacteria that randomly develop mutations that happen to protect the cell against antibiotics are the ones that will survive the drug. They live on to reproduce and spread their resistant genes throughout the population. And since a bacterium can reproduce a new generation in just minutes, you can see how resistance can spread quickly.

The first resistance strategy is to block the ability of the drug to penetrate the bacterial cell at all. This can be accomplished by increasing the thickness of the cell wall or by changing the size of the pores in the cell membrane. Another way of accomplishing this same strategy is to produce a pumping mechanism, which will spit the drug out from the cell.

The second major drug resistance strategy is to change the target molecule for the drug. A mutated protein produced MRSA, and a change in the structure of the cell wall material gave us VRSA. The antibiotic stops working because it can no longer bind to its target molecule.

The third and final bacterial strategy to avoid drugs is enzymatic inactivation. The bacterium develops the ability to inactivate the drug by producing enzymes that chop it up or block its activity. Bacteria that make these enzymes may actually also protect nonresistant bacteria in their locale by neutralizing the drug as it arrives in the area.

# Solving the Drug Resistance Problem

There's no easy answer to the problem of drug-resistant bacteria. Bacteria existed long, long before humans — and they'll exist long after humans vanish from this planet. They simply adapt and evolve to protect themselves against the chemicals we use — a process that happens very quickly. At the same time that we have created antibiotic-resistant germs, we have become as a society so dependent on antimicrobics that we can't easily simply stop their use. We also have an increasing population of people with compromised immune systems. People with HIV/AIDS, transplanted organs, or autoimmune diseases such as lupus and rheumatoid arthritis often need to take regular, low doses of antibiotics over long periods of time. Prophylactic doses of antibiotics help prevent infection in these people, which is good, but the practice also allows bacteria and viruses to multiply while exposed to low concentrations of these drugs. This only encourages the development of more and more resistance genes.

If it were possible to stop the use of antimicrobics all together, bacteria and viruses would slowly revert to their previous, less resistant forms. It is energy intensive to carry DNA that isn't useful. If the resistance genes no longer provide a selective advantage to the bacteria, over time these genes will be lost. Today, awareness of the antibiotic resistance problem is growing. Physicians' guidelines now emphasize the appropriate use of antibiotics. Many HMOs now have policies that say their doctors will prescribe antibiotics only when they are certain the illness is caused by a bacterium, not a virus. Hospitals are paying increasing attention to avoiding infection to begin with through better procedures that help prevent transmission of germs, especially MRSA.

## Resistant Malaria

Drug resistance isn't confined to antibiotics that kill bacteria. Malaria, the most common fatal infectious disease in the world, is also now drug resistant.

Current estimates are that between one and two million people die every year from malaria. Many researchers feel that if all the indirect damages of malaria were calculated, the disease would cause half of all human deaths every year globally.

Malaria is caused by a protozoan parasite that is transmitted by mosquitoes. Because tropical areas of the globe support mosquito populations year round, malaria is a disease against which millions of humans must take preventative drugs daily. The malaria parasite has developed resistance against virtually every one of these drugs—and multidrug-resistant malaria is a disease against which there are no easy answers. Because the parasite changes its form in the human, effective vaccines for malaria prevention are very hard to make. Despite much research, there has been little progress in this area. New drugs to fight malaria are in development, but here too it is only a matter of time before resistance develops. Prevention, particularly through the use of insecticide-treated mosquito nets, is the most effective approach for now.

## The Dirt Factor

We create untreatable superbugs when we oversanitize with antimicrobial cleansers and overmedicate with antibiotic drugs. We look for the quick fix that will supposedly keep us safe from deadly germs, but there isn't one. Every infection that you suffer through in the short term makes you stronger in the long term, and eventually your body will have all the skills it needs to keep you healthy regardless of your environment. There is never a substitute for hard work: Your immunity depends upon it every bit as much as your diet, your education, your job, your happiness. There is no magic pill that will protect you as well as your fully equipped immunological army.

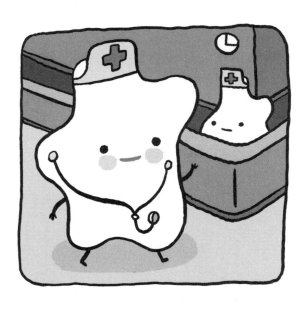

## RULE 4:

# Immunity the Easy Way: Keep Your Vaccinations Up to Date

You might think that with my apparent "let Mother Nature take her course" philosophy, I would oppose vaccination. Absolutely not. My recommendation of vaccinations goes along with my "dirt is good" argument. A little exposure, under the right circumstances, is a good thing.

The diseases against which successful vaccination campaigns have been mounted have in common that they were highly dangerous or fatal in their natural state. Individuals who survived these diseases developed strong natural immunity, but many people did not survive, or if they did, had permanent disabilities such as blindness or paralysis.

One of the greatest scientific achievements of the 20th century was the development of vaccinations against diseases that killed millions in previous centuries. Because of widespread vaccination, diseases such as diphtheria, smallpox, measles, and polio today are very rare in the developed world. Vaccination against smallpox has been around for centuries, but it wasn't until 1980, following a massive international vaccination effort, that smallpox became the first—and so far the only—human disease to become extinct. Massive vaccination programs in the 1950s and 1960s brought immunization against polio to the United States, ending the polio epidemics that swept the country earlier in the century. Although polio remains a problem in a few countries, such as Nigeria, in the United States and most of the world this crippling disease has been vanquished.

Vaccines today are generally forms of the bacterium or virus that have been altered so that they can't cause disease, but still produce a strong immune response. That means vaccinations are simply an artificial way to enhance your natural immune response. That's far preferable to actually getting a possibly fatal disease such as bacterial meningitis. The immunity from a vaccine is usually long lasting and effective. Unlike antimicrobics and antiseptics, vaccines don't encourage the selection of mutant, more dangerous organisms. Instead, a vaccine pumps up your own immune response so it is better able to protect you. Vaccines work in tandem with Mother Nature, not in opposition to her.

Today's vaccines are extremely safe and extremely effective: To avoid them is to play roulette with your health.

## What's in a Vaccine?

Vaccines are inoculations incorporating a killed, weakened, or even living microbe. The antigens in the inoculation stimulate the formation of immunity against whatever disease agent is in the vaccine. (The word *inoculation* is a quick way of saying "introduction into the body of the causative agent of a disease.") When you receive a vaccination, you are receiving an injection (usually—some vaccines are administered nasally or orally) of a harmless version of a dangerous germ. In the case of vaccines against bacterial diseases, the vaccine often contains an inactivated version of the bacterial toxin called a toxoid. This is true of the vaccines against diphtheria, tetanus, and pertussis (whooping cough). Because these vaccines contain only a neutralized protein product of the bacterium, there is no possibility of getting an infection from the inoculation, because there's nothing in the vaccine that produces more of the toxoid. Your body simply responds to the stimulation from the toxoid by producing an antibody against it. As your body produces the antibody, memory cells are produced. These cells will stay on watch for many years to come, waiting for the real disease agent to try to enter your body. If this happens, they will very quickly produce the antibodies that will neutralize the toxin, which will prevent you from becoming ill. The whole process will happen so quickly and effectively that you'll never know you were under attack from a killer germ.

Other antibacterial vaccines, such as those for *Haemophilus influenzae* and *Streptococcus pneumoniae*, which are both causes of life-threatening meningitis in children, include the capsule material that covers the bacterium and a protein from the bacterium to stimulate the production of specific IgA antibodies. The vaccine creates long-lived memory cells in the mucosal surfaces, such as those lining your nose, which will produce antibodies to keep the bacteria from penetrating that barrier.

Vaccines against viral diseases come in three categories: killed, live-attenuated, and component. The Salk polio vaccine is an example of a killed viral vaccine. Your immune system responds to a protein in the vaccine by making an antibody that would prevent the living virus, if you were ever to encounter it, from being able to attach to and infect a cell. The measles, mumps, and rubella vaccine (called MMR for short) is an example of a live-attenuated vaccine. In this vaccine, each of the three viruses has been altered so that it can't cause disease but can still stimulate immunity. This type of vaccine causes the production of both antibody and cell-mediated immunity. When you get the MMR vaccine, your immune system is stimulated by the whole life cycle of the viruses. But because the viruses have been altered to be very weak, they're nowhere near as dangerous as the "wild type" virus found in the environment. That means you get the benefit of immunity against the wild type virus without ever having to get sick from it. The final type of antivirus vaccine is the component vaccine, exemplified by the hepatitis B vaccine and the new human papillomavirus vaccine (Gardasil). In these vaccines, a single molecule of the virus, chosen specifically because it's a strong target for immunity, is created in the laboratory using recombinant DNA technology. Just the antigen, not the whole virus, becomes the vaccine. Your body responds to this one antigen by making antibodies against it.

Because viruses are intracellular agents, when we grow them in the laboratory we have to grow them inside living cells. Viruses are often grown inside hen's eggs, so persons who are allergic to eggs may have reactions to the MMR, influenza, and yellow fever vaccines. This is why you will be asked about egg allergies before you receive one of these inoculations. It's not because the virus material is dangerous but because if you are allergic to eggs, it's dangerous to be exposed to egg proteins by injection.

Some vaccines are mixed with an adjuvant, a harmless substance that is included as a way of increasing the speed and intensity of the immune response. Because most vaccine constituents have been altered so they can't multiply in your body, and because your immune response multiplies in response to the multiplication of an invader, adjuvants work to amplify your immune response. Adjuvants often increase inflammation at the injection site—and inflammation is essential to calling in white blood cells and getting the whole immune response ball rolling. The presence of an adjuvant is why you will sometimes experience minor swelling, redness, heat, and pain at the injection site. It's the evidence that your immune response is doing its job and that you are making a healthy response to the vaccine.

# Vaccines for Everyone

Vaccines are often thought of as a childhood thing—you have to go get your shots and you get a lollipop on the way out. Of course, most vaccines are given to kids to help them avoid dangerous illnesses as early as possible, but there are also vaccines that teens, adults, and older adults should routinely get.

According to the Centers for Disease Control, kids should get the hepatitis B vaccine at birth. At two months, they should get the first shots of vaccines for combined diphtheria, tetanus, pertussis (DTaP), *Haemophilus influenzae* (Hib), pneumococcus, and polio. At the age of 12 months, the baby should get the vaccines for measles, mumps, and rubella (MMR), varicella (chicken pox), and hepatitis A. Older kids (11 and up) should get the vaccine for human papillomavirus (HPV) and the meningococcal vaccine. The human papillomavirus vaccine provides very strong protection against the formation of genital warts. Among those vaccinated in the United States, it should prevent at least 50 percent of the cases of cervical cancer. Right now, there are over 11,000 new cases every year of this preventable cancer; 4,000 women die from it every year. Cutting those numbers in half will be a big improvement.

Flu shots every year are a good idea for everyone of any age, including babies (they can get a nasal version). While the vaccine may not fully protect every individual, overall it's quite effective at preventing a highly contagious illness that can leave you sneezing, coughing, and feeling extremely lousy for a week or longer. The influenza vaccine is formulated yearly based on our best guesses of what strains of virus will be most common worldwide. Influenza virus is an example of a family of viruses that is capable of drastic genetic changes when animal influenza viruses and human influenza viruses end up infecting a single cell. This can typically happen in eastern Asia, where large populations of animals and humans live together in crowded conditions. Perhaps you remember our recent concerns about swine flu and bird flu. These were illnesses where new viruses arose (or were feared to be arising) from combinations of swine or bird influenza viruses with human strains. So, every year, the scientific community tries to anticipate which changes to the flu vaccine are needed—an imperfect system to be sure, but trying to predict the future is always an imperfect art.

The CDC also suggests that older adults (over age 60), anyone with a chronic disease such as type 1 diabetes or emphysema, and anyone with a compromised immune system should get an annual pneumococcal vaccine to prevent bacterial pneumonia.

In 2006, a vaccine for shingles (also known as *Herpes zoster*) became available. Shingles is a very painful skin rash that affects mostly adults over age 50 and can have serious complications. It's caused by the same virus that causes chickenpox. If you've ever had chickenpox, the virus stays dormant in your body, hiding out harmlessly in your nerve cells. The chickenpox vaccine virus won't cause shingles, so only persons who have had real chickenpox and are therefore infected with the dormant virulent virus will be at risk for developing shingles. If your immune system becomes weakened (by aging, illness, chemotherapy, and many other possible causes), the virus can become active again, causing shingles. The new vaccine is recommended for adults over age 60. It's effective in preventing shingles completely about 50 percent of the time. People who get the shot and still get the disease usually have a milder case with less pain.

# To Vaccinate or Not to Vaccinate: NOT EVEN A QUESTION!

Some parents are so terrified by sensational media reports linking childhood vaccines to horrifying conditions and crippling side effects that they refuse to vaccinate their children.

For any of the usual childhood vaccines, there is no credible scientific evidence that any of this is true. One of the most pervasive urban legends links MMR vaccination to autism. This false belief and others like it cause a small population of parents to forego vaccinating their children. The predictable outcome is outbreaks of life-threatening diseases in these unprotected children.

The MMR vaccine was introduced in the late 1980s. At roughly the same time, for unclear reasons, the number of children diagnosed with autism started to rise. Most children get their first MMR shot when they're around a year old and then get a second shot when they start school, usually between the ages of four and six—the same ages when children with autism are often diagnosed. Researchers seeking a reason for the rise in autism cases looked at a possible link between the MMR vaccine and autism. A study in 1998 claimed there was such a link, but the methodology of the paper was so flawed that it was soon discredited.

Since then, researchers have shown, in numerous carefully designed scientific studies reported in major medical journals, that there is no logical link between autism and the MMR vaccination—and also no connection between autism and thimerosal, a preservative used in the vaccine. For example, there is no difference in the age at diagnosis of autism in vaccinated versus unvaccinated children, and there is no relationship between the onset of regressive symptoms of autism and getting the vaccine. The rate of autism didn't drop after 1999, when thimerosal was removed from the vaccine. According to some sources, the diagnosis of autism spectrum disorders increased by 373 percent between 1980 and 1994, even though vaccination rates in children remained relatively constant.

If you want to assign a cause-and-effect relationship between autism and anything, you would have to find some other variable in our environment that has increased by the same proportion during this time frame. So far, no one has. The truth is that we don't understand what causes autism. It's likely that the increased rate of diagnosis is multifactorial, perhaps involving environmental stimuli and genetic vulnerabilities, and due at least in part to the increased sensitivity of our modern diagnostic tests and changes in the diagnostic guidelines.

## The Last Word on MMR Safety

A major study in 2008, published in the prestigious *Public Library of Science*, firmly refutes any possible link between MMR vaccination and autism. The study used DNA analysis to look for the presence of genetic material from the measles vaccine in kids who were recently diagnosed with autism. The analysis showed that the virus was present in only one of the 25 autistic children studied—and in only one of the control group of 13 children without autism. In addition, the study found no connection between the timing of receiving the vaccine and the onset of gastrointestinal symptoms associated with autism.

Over the past couple of decades, more than 20 epidemiological studies have failed to show a link between autism and the MMR vaccine. This latest study should be the last word on the subject.

Other unfounded fears about vaccination simply show the power of anecdotes and outdated information over hard facts. For example, some parents don't want their child to receive the pertussis (whooping cough) vaccine because they fear serious side effects. In fact, the older pertussis vaccine could cause temporary side effects, including a high fever in about one out of every 330 doses. In the 1970s, concerns about the side effects were so widespread that some countries stopped using the vaccine. In Japan, for instance, the pertussis vaccine was dropped in 1975. In the three years before that, there were 400 cases of pertussis and 10 deaths in all of Japan. In the three years after the vaccine was halted, there were 13,000 cases of pertussis and 113 deaths. Pretty clearly, the risk of temporary side effects from the vaccine far outweighed the risk of not giving it, and Japan went back to pertussis vaccination. Similar situations happened in England, Sweden, and elsewhere. After seeing dangerous spikes in the number of whooping cough cases, these countries all went back to routine vaccination.

This story is a good example not only of how the benefits of vaccines outweigh the risks, it's also a good example of how outdated information still floats around. The older version of the pertussis vaccine has been replaced by a newer version that is just as effective but has a much lower risk of side effects.

Another issue that's often raised by anti-vaccine proponents on their websites and in distorted media reports is whether vaccines are really needed at all. Of course they are, as the pertussis story shows. The problem here is that widespread vaccination programs have been so successful that most parents today have no idea how dangerous childhood diseases can actually be.

Measles, for instance, is a rare illness in the United States today, because the vast majority of kids are immunized against it. But the virus is still out there, and it's highly contagious. If you don't immunize your child, at some point he is likely to encounter the wild type virus and get sick from it. In addition, the measles vaccine isn't as widely used as it should be in some other countries, so an unimmunized person who travels to one of these countries — or stays home and encounters a person from one of those countries — will have a very good chance of catching the disease.

Another good reason to get immunized is to protect the people around you. Someone who's not immunized against measles can infect a baby who hasn't had the MMR vaccine yet, for instance.

There's a tendency to think of diseases such as measles as childhood problems that kids get over quickly and easily. That's not always the case. With measles, for instance, six in a hundred kids will get pneumonia, one in a thousand will get encephalitis (inflammation of the brain), and two in a thousand will die. Compare that to the risk of severe allergic reaction to the MMR vaccine: one in a million.

Similar issues arise with the hepatitis B vaccine. Parents wonder if the shot is needed at all, because hepatitis B is most often transmitted from a mother to a baby. If the mother doesn't have the disease, why does the baby need the vaccination? The baby still does, because hepatitis B is very widespread. The disease can be passed on to a child by any infected person — another family member, someone at school or day care, a playmate.

Worldwide, about 375 million people are infected with the hepatitis B virus. Lifelong infection with the virus causes liver disease and liver cancer — a million people a year die from it. In the United States, about 12.5 million people have been infected with hepatitis B, and about 5,000 die from it each year (far more than die of all other vaccine-preventable diseases put together). When babies and young children get hepatitis B, they're at lifelong risk of developing severe liver disease. In fact, 25 percent of kids infected with hepatitis B will die of liver-related disease in adulthood. The illness often doesn't produce noticeable symptoms at first — the liver problems take decades of infection to develop.

Since routine hepatitis B vaccination began in the 1980s, the number of new cases among kids has declined markedly. That in turn leads to a long-term decline in the incidence — and huge social and financial cost—of debilitating liver disease and death related to the virus.

There is, by the way, no truth to the sensational media accounts supposedly linking the hepatitis B vaccine to sudden infant death syndrome (SIDS) or arthritis, multiple sclerosis, and vaguely defined neurological problems. (There's also absolutely no truth to the rumor that the polio vaccine is the cause of AIDS.)

Another common parental objection to all those shots a baby has to get is that it just can't be good for the little tyke to get so many vaccines before he's even a year old—or even on his first day of life for the hepatitis B vaccine. This is another myth that I hope this book will help dispel. If you've read to this point, you know that the immune system of even a newborn is already actively fending off infections and is capable of a robust immune response. Vaccines are just one more thing out of many for the baby's immune system to respond to—and respond it will, quickly and thoroughly.

The advantage of giving kids several vaccines at once is twofold. First, it immunizes the kids against as many illnesses as possible as quickly as possible. Second, it saves a lot of parental time and energy to have just one visit to the pediatrician for combined vaccines instead of several visits for individual vaccines.

Another myth I want to dispel is the idea that getting a natural infection is somehow "healthier" than being immunized. OK, it's true that getting diphtheria, if you manage to live through it, will quickly give you strong immunity, while it takes at least three diphtheria shots over several years to give comparable immunity. The risk of permanent injury or even death from diphtheria is very high, however, while the risks of the shots are extremely low. Common sense says get the shots.

## The Dirt Factor

When dirt means exposure to dangerous diseases such as polio, tetanus, diphtheria, and measles, it's clearly not good. You don't want to build up your immune system by exposure to germs that could kill or cripple you. Fortunately, in the modern world many of the deadly diseases of the past are now very rare. Because we have effective sewage treatment and a very safe water supply, epidemics of illnesses such as cholera are almost unheard of in the developed world. Likewise, extensive vaccination programs have nearly eliminated dangerous illnesses like measles.

Your immune system needs dirt to develop and stay strong, but giving it a little help is just fine. Vaccination gives you immunity without illness; sanitation helps you avoid illnesses that can overwhelm even the strongest of immune systems. Between the two, you have less to fear from dirt than ever before in history.

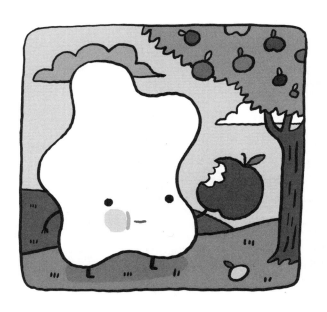

# RULE 5:

# Always Ask First, What Would Mother Nature Do? Common Sense as a Cure

Today many of us rush to the drugstore the moment we get sick with something that causes a runny nose, a cough, an upset stomach, a headache. We depend on quick pharmaceutical fixes that mask the symptoms instead of listening to the symptoms of our illness and doing what they tell us: rest, drink plenty of fluids, and let your immune system do its job.

Drugs, both prescription and over-the-counter, can help us avoid some discomfort, but too often we become dependent on them. In general, drugs to treat symptoms do nothing to protect us from the need for their repeated use in the future—and may not even really help with the symptoms anyway. Antibiotics and other antimicrobial drugs may sometimes be medically appropriate, but relying on them for anything less than a serious illness or infection does nothing to strengthen your immunity and help you avoid the need for them in the future. Relying instead on your immune system usually works very well, and will work for you even better in the future. Your immune system becomes stronger with each exposure to a germ.

If you want to live a long, healthy life, there's no substitute for immunologic exercise, starting in infancy. White blood cells multiply in response to a challenge: Each exposure to a germ gives your immune system more memory cells, which means you can respond faster and more aggressively the next time that particular germ tries to attack. It will be stopped in its tracks so quickly and efficiently that you probably won't even notice. A rapid immune response means you won't have any symptoms, which means you won't need to medicate yourself, much less take antimicrobial drugs.

What we need is a return to common sense. Very little in life that is worthwhile comes without effort, and your immunity is no exception. A healthy immune system comes in part from healthy living. Just as lifestyle changes, not a quick-fix diet, are needed for successful weight control, your immune system functions best when you give your body the rest and nutrition it needs.

# Listening to Your Body

Modern life is a constant balancing act between work and leisure, job and family, health and illness. Many decisions are forced upon us by circumstances that are unavoidable, but the quality of your life can definitely be improved if you stop to listen to what your body is telling you.

Inflammation is your body's first response to an injury or attack by an invader. The affected area gets red, swollen, hot, and painful. Although we spend a tremendous amount of money as a society on relieving the unpleasant manifestations of the inflammatory process, inflammation is the essential first step in the development of your immune response. It sets the immune cascade in motion.

Inflammation is so critical to the immunologic response because it calls in the appropriate white blood cells to fight infection and begin tissue repair. Do you treat it with drugs (prescription or over-the-counter) that will reduce the inflammation, or do you realize that inflammation is Mother Nature's way of telling you to take it easy and allow your body the rest it needs to heal itself? The first choice numbs you to the injury or illness and allows you to continue the use of that tissue, possibly to the point of doing permanent harm. The second choice results in a stronger, healthier tissue that will resist this injury or illness in the future.

# What Would Mother Nature Do?

When your immune system is busy fighting off invaders, it needs a lot of your body's resources. By staying home and taking it easy, you let your body divert more of its nutrients and energy to your immune system. That's simple common sense for your own health, and it also has important implications for the health of others. Is it really a good idea, for example, to drag your sneezing, coughing, grouchy body to the office when you have a cold or flu? Mother Nature would tell you to stay home, keep your germs to yourself, and let your immune system do its work and kill off the virus that much more quickly. The viruses that cause colds, however, think otherwise. Instead of making you so sick you have to stay in bed, they make you just sick enough that you can manage to get to work. That's exactly what the virus wants, because it needs new hosts to continue to survive. Every time you sneeze, cough, or touch something, you're helping the virus spread itself to other victims. Stay home instead and let your immune system teach the virus who's boss.

Often the unpleasant symptoms of an illness, annoying as they may be, are your body's way of evicting the invaders. When you cough from the flu or a cold, for instance, you're mechanically expelling some of the virus from your body. That's what the virus wants, because it needs to find more people to infect. Here's where common sense comes in. Since you're coughing up virus-laden mucus and saliva, avoid passing the bug to others by staying home and using good sanitation (lots of clean tissues, for instance) to try to keep from infecting family members. Logic also tells you that there's a reason you're sneezing and have a runny nose—all that mucus is your body's way of kicking the virus out. When you dose yourself with over-the-counter cough medicines and decongestants, you're interfering with your healing process. You may feel temporarily better (leaving aside the dangerous drowsiness and cross-reactions these drugs can cause), but you'll probably be sicker longer.

Follow Mother Nature's treatment plan instead: stay home, rest, and drink plenty of fluids to replace what you're losing and help keep your mucus thin and easy to expel.

## Cold Medications and Kids

Cold medications only mask symptoms—they don't do anything to help you get over the cold faster. And when it comes to kids, cold medications can be downright dangerous.

According to the Centers for Disease Control, every year some 11,000 kids aged 11 and younger end up in the emergency room after taking cold and cough medicines. The Food and Drug Administration (FDA) says these drugs shouldn't be given to children under age two—and the agency is currently reassessing whether these drugs are really safe for older children. Steam from a humidifier, saline drops, and a bulb syringe can help relieve nasal congestion in babies. Plenty of fluids and a quiet environment that encourages rest will help the baby get over the cold on her own, without drugs.

It's tough on you as a parent to deal with a sick, fussy baby, but remember, the cold your child conquers today is the cold he or she won't get later on.

Obviously, taking an antibiotic won't help with the viruses that cause colds, flu, and sore throats (only about 15 percent of sore throats are caused by the bacterium *Streptococcus*). Recent research has shown that antibiotics also don't help sinusitis, even when it's caused by a bacterium. In fact, antibiotics such as amoxicillin are no better at cutting short a sinus infection than a placebo.

What about antiviral drugs for the flu? Oseltamivir (Tamiflu) and similar drugs are sometimes prescribed to treat or prevent the flu. They are used mostly for people with compromised immunity or chronic health problems that can't get a flu shot. They're also used to prevent and treat flu outbreaks in nursing homes and other shared-living facilities. For these people, a case of the flu could cause very serious illness or even death.

For the rest of us, taking oseltamivir or another antiviral drug usually isn't necessary. The drug only works if you take it within 12 to 48 hours of the onset of symptoms. If taken in time, it may help lessen the symptoms, but it probably won't shorten the duration of the illness. Given the realities of our health-care system, most people won't get to a doctor and be diagnosed with flu in time for the drug to be helpful. More importantly, just as inappropriate use of antibiotics causes resistance in bacteria, antiviral drugs cause resistance in viruses, even one that mutates as quickly as the flu virus. An older antiviral flu drug, amantadine (Symmetrel), causes near 100 percent resistance in the flu virus, which is why today it's rarely prescribed. While an antiviral drug might just make you feel a little better, it comes at a cost in dollars and public health. The price isn't worth the very limited benefit and potential risks.

Taking drugs to stop the symptoms of an upset stomach or diarrhea from an illness is usually counterproductive and could even be dangerous. In fact, doctors usually advise against it. Most cases of diarrhea will go away on their own in two to three days without any medical treatment. Often a "stomach flu" is caused by a virus, in which case antibiotics are useless. When diarrhea is caused by one of the common food-poisoning bacteria, such as *Salmonella* or *E. coli,* antibiotics may actually be harmful.

When you have diarrhea, your body is eliminating both the causative germ and the toxins it produces — in fact, the toxins, not the germs themselves, may be the cause of the diarrhea. As with a cold, this is the germ's way of getting out of your body to infect someone else. Let it. When you take antidiarrheal drugs, you're just keeping the toxins and germs from passing out of your body, while the drugs might well make you sicker. Apply common sense instead. Your own immune system can take care of the germs left behind, and staying home and practicing good hygiene can help keep the germs from being passed on. Drink plenty of fluids to keep from getting dehydrated, and stick to a bland diet until your bowels return to normal. Ditto for "stomach bugs" and "food poisoning" that make you vomit. You want to get the germs and their toxins out of your system, and throwing up is a pretty effective way to do it. The important thing usually isn't to stop the vomiting; it's to avoid dehydration by drinking plenty of fluids.

# Stress and Immunity

You've probably noticed that you tend to get sick when you've gone through a period of high stress, excessive work, or when you haven't been getting much sleep. You get sick because all that stress has a negative effect on your immune system.

We tend to use the word *stress* pretty loosely these days, saying that anything from a mild annoyance to a major traumatic event is stressful. From your body's point of view, however, stress has a more specific meaning. It falls into two categories: acute and chronic.

Acute stress happens all at once: You have a close call while driving, for instance, or you have a brief confrontation with someone. Your heart pounds, your blood pressure rises, and then the incident is over. Your body quickly returns to normal. Chronic stress is stress that is ongoing and inescapable. It could be from a job you hate, or from being in a bad relationship, or from the demands of caring for someone who's ill. In fact, it could be simply from trying to juggle family life, work, and all the other demands of modern living. Any situation that makes never-ending demands over a long time will cause chronic stress. This is the sort of stress that can damage your immune system.

Your body reacts to an episode of acute stress by triggering your natural "fight or flight" response. In earlier times, when you were threatened by a saber-toothed cat, you had to make a snap decision: attack the cat with your spear or run away from it as fast as you can. To help you throw the spear harder or run faster, your body releases stress hormones, such as epinephrine, that speed up your heart rate, slow your digestion, increase the blood flow to your arms and legs, and overall give you a burst of energy and strength. If you're also lucky, you survive to hunt another day.

Today's world is less dangerous but more complex. We still experience acute stress, but we also have levels of chronic stress cavemen never experienced—and that our bodies aren't really adapted to withstand. Constant exposure to elevated levels of stress hormones, particularly one called cortisol, makes bad things happen to your immune system. The stress hormones tell your immune system cells to stop fighting so your body can divert its resources elsewhere. Your immune system's response becomes blunted and you become more likely to get sick. Making the situation worse is that people coping with chronic stress often can't make good lifestyle choices. They don't eat well or get enough sleep, which only suppresses the immune system even more.

Stuff happens in life—there are no easy solutions to chronic stress, but those with the strongest immune systems will be less affected immunologically. Of course, even people who have strong, well-trained immune systems will still experience immune suppression from chronic stress. The difference is that the effect may take a little longer to kick in for them, and they may return to normal faster.

## The Dirt Factor

Mother Nature has given you all the elements to build a strong immune system, but you have to put it into action and take care of it. A strong immune system gets built up by plenty of exercise — that's why you need a lifetime of exposure to plenty of dirt. Your healthy immune system is your savings account for a healthy retirement. If you constantly make withdrawals and live with a negative health balance due to too much stress, too little rest, and too many chemicals, you will arrive at a point where you have no reserves for any catastrophic illness that might lurk in your future.

A healthy lifestyle and a healthy immune system also help lessen the impact of the inevitable decline in immunity that comes with advancing age. If you've built up a large balance in your health account, you'll still have plenty left even after the withdrawals that come with age. A lifestyle that gives you the food, rest, exercise, and other elements you need for basic good health contributes to a healthy immune response and increases the likelihood of a long, productive life.

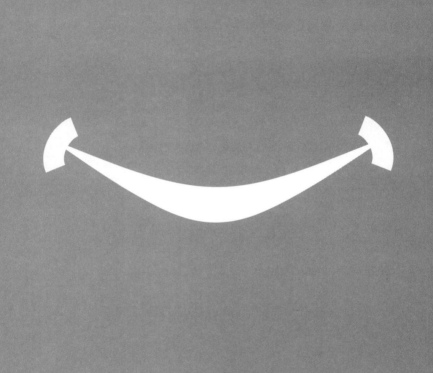

# Glossary

-------------

# Glossary

**Abscess.** A collection of dead and dying bacteria and dead and dying neutrophils (pus) that forms to wall off an area of your body that has been invaded.

**Active immunity.** Immunity achieved by exposure to a germ and the activation of your white blood cells to destroy the invader, multiply, and produce "memory" of the invasion, which will cause any future immune response to be stronger, faster, and more efficient.

**Adjuvant.** A material injected along with a vaccine to make the immune response happen faster and stronger than it would have otherwise. It is believed that adjuvants act to increase nonspecific inflammation so that white blood cells become activated more efficiently.

**Allergen.** A molecule against which you make an allergic response.

**Allergy.** An immune response in which IgE antibody is made against something in your environment, and degranulating mast cells and basophils cause you to damage your own tissues. An allergic response is an antiparasite response misdirected against something harmless in your environment, like dust, pollen, or animal dander.

**Anatomical barriers.** The systems of your body that act to stop germs from getting inside you. They include the skin and mucous membranes.

**Angry macrophage.** A macrophage that has been stimulated by the soluble mediators (cytokines) of a T helper 1 cell so that it becomes better at the job of killing what it has eaten.

**Antibacterial.** A drug or chemical that inhibits or kills bacteria.

**Antibiotic.** Classically, a chemical produced by one microbe that impedes the growth and development of another. It is now used more broadly to mean any drug used to combat bacterial infections, regardless of whether that drug has been derived from another microbe or has been artificially synthesized in a laboratory.

**Antibody.** A protein secretion of B lymphocytes and plasma cells that circulates in your bloodstream and has specificity for particular germs. Antibodies may prevent the binding of harmful invaders to your cells, assist the phagocytosis of your phagocytic cells, or activate complement to cause a germ to dissolve.

**Antibody-dependent cell-mediated cytotoxicity (ADCC).** The form of extracellular killing of germs that may be done by neutrophils, monocytes, eosinophils, and natural killer cells. An IgG antibody molecule binds to a receptor on the surface of a white blood cell after binding specifically to the surface of the invader. The white blood cell then releases toxic chemicals that cause the germ to be killed extracellularly.

**Antifungal.** A chemical or drug that inhibits or kills fungi (molds).

**Antigen.** Any foreign substance, such as molecules on the surface of a bacterium or virus that stimulates an immune response using antibodies.

**Antimicrobic.** A chemical or drug that inhibits or kills any microbe (microscopic organism), which may include viruses, bacteria, fungi, or protozoa (single-celled parasites).

**Antiparasitic.** A chemical or drug that inhibits or kills parasites, which may include single-celled parasites (protozoa) or multicellular worms (helminths).

**Antitoxin antibodies.** Antibodies made in response to the toxic protein secretions of some bacteria.

**Antiviral.** A chemical or drug that inhibits or kills viruses.

**Atopic/atopy.** An atopic individual is one who mounts harmful allergic responses against things which are harmless in their environment. Atopy is the state of being allergic.

**Autoantibodies.** Antibodies that bind to and damage one's own cells or tissues.

**Autoimmunity.** The state of mounting an immune response against one's own cells or tissues.

**B cell.** The subcategory of lymphocytes that produce antibody molecules and are the precursor of the plasma cell, whose job it is to pump antibodies into the circulation.

**Bacteria.** Single-celled life-forms that are much smaller than our cells, lack a nucleus, and reproduce themselves asexually by a process of division into two (binary fission).

**Bacteriophage.** A virus that infects bacteria.

**Basophil.** A white blood cell that contains granules of toxic chemicals designed to be dumped on parasites when they try to penetrate your body. When basophils direct their action toward harmless environmental materials, allergy results. Basophils differentiate into mast cells when they leave the circulation and go to live in the tissues under the skin and mucosa.

**Binary fission.** The asexual process of division into two. The means by which bacteria make more bacteria.

**Capsule.** A slimy covering over some bacteria and fungi that makes it difficult for phagocytes to grab them.

**Cell-mediated immunity.** The arm of your immune response meant to identify cells of your body altered either by cancerous change or by an infectious process happening inside them. It is masterminded by Th1 lymphocytes; the killer cells include macrophages, cytotoxic T lymphocytes, and natural killer cells.

**Cellular barriers.** The cells lining the surfaces of your body (both internal and external) that attempt to stop the penetration of germs. Most of these cells are phagocytic and will eat and digest foreign invaders.

**Chemical barriers.** The chemicals produced by your body to stop the invasion of germs. Your stomach is very acidic and will dissolve most things that enter. Your saliva and tears contain chemicals which dissolve the cell walls of bacteria, and your skin is also acidic to stop the growth of invaders.

**Chromosome.** A large molecule of double-stranded DNA that contains the genes that encode the proteins necessary for life.

**Class I MHC.** A set of molecules found on the surface of your cells, inherited from each of your parents, that define you as a unique being.

**Class II MHC.** A set of molecules found on the surface of your immune cells, inherited from each of your parents, that present foreign proteins to your T lymphocytes for immunologic recognition.

**Clone.** A group of cells with identical characteristics produced by the division of a single progenitor cell.

**Complement.** A set of proteins that circulate in the body and activate one another in a cascading fashion to dissolve particles, including pathogens, to which they become attached.

**Component vaccine.** A viral vaccine composed of only one component of the virus. For example, the hepatitis B vaccine is a single molecule, the surface protein of the virus, created in the laboratory by recombinant DNA technology. The vaccine against human papillomavirus is made of the shell of the four most common strains of that virus, again produced by recombinant DNA technology.

**Constant domain.** The relatively uniform areas of the antibody molecule that make up the tail of the Y-shaped molecule and give the antibody molecule its function.

**CTL.** See cytotoxic T lymphocyte.

**Cytokine.** A soluble product of one cell that is used to communicate with other cells.

**Cytotoxic T lymphocyte (CTL).** A T lymphocyte that identifies changes in the surfaces of one's own cells that are associated with disease processes, and kills the cell(s) that are abnormal. They are the most important protective response against viruses and many cancers.

**Dimer**. A molecule made of two identical halves, such as secretory IgA, which is composed of two Y-shaped monomers held together by a single joining chain.

**Disinfectant.** A chemical that removes disease-causing germs from an area.

**DNA (deoxyribonucleic acid).** The genetic material of life. This is the material arranged into the genes and chromosomes that make every individual unique.

**DPT vaccine.** The childhood vaccine against diphtheria, pertussis (whooping cough), and tetanus. It consists of the inactivated protein toxin from each of these bacteria that cause life-threatening diseases in young children.

**Drug resistance.** The ability of microorganisms to resist inhibition or killing by the drugs we use to treat them.

**Eosinophil.** A granular white blood cell that contains materials toxic to worm parasites. This cell is attracted to areas where parasites have penetrated the skin or mucous membranes, and dumps its toxic contents on the immature worms to attempt to kill them. When parasites are not common in a society, eosinophils are attracted to areas of allergic hypersensitivity.

**Epithelial cells.** Cells that line or cover surfaces of your body, such as your mouth, nose, throat, eyes, and intestines.

**Eustachian tubes.** The internal openings of the inner ear.

**Extracellular.** Outside of a cell. In the case of a germ, one that lives outside your cells, such as most bacteria, most fungi, and most parasites.

**Fungi.** A group of organisms including yeasts, molds, and mushrooms, that may be single celled or multicellular and contain a complex carbohydrate cell wall.

**Gene pool.** The complete set of unique genetic traits available to a species or population of organisms.

**Genetic variant.** A member of a species that has a different genetic makeup from another member of the same species. For example, blue eyes and brown eyes are genetic variants of eye color genes.

**Genome.** The genetic makeup of an organism.

**Granulocyte.** A white blood cell that contains granules in its cytoplasm. These include neutrophils, basophils, and eosinophils.

**Helper T (Th) cell.** A lymphocyte selected in the thymus that serves to regulate the immune response. These cells produce the cytokines that cause all the other cells of your immune response to multiply and become activated.

***Hemophilus influenzae* vaccine (H-flu vaccine).** A vaccine for infants that contains the capsular material of this bacterium, which can cause a life-threatening meningitis in children between three months and two years of age.

**Human immunodeficiency virus (HIV).** The virus in the retrovirus family that causes acquired immunodeficiency syndrome (AIDS) by infecting helper T cells and macrophages.

**IgA (immunoglobulin A).** The principal antibody of the mucosal surfaces of the body that prevents germs from adhering in those locations.

**IgE (immunoglobulin E).** The antibody that binds to the receptors on mast cells, basophils, and eosinophils and "aims" the release of the toxic granules onto parasites or allergens.

**IgG (immunoglobulin G).** The most common class of antibody made after initial exposure. It is capable of opsonization, activation of complement, and is pumped across the placenta to protect a fetus in the womb.

**IgM (immunoglobulin M).** The first antibody made in response to any infection, it is made of five Y-shaped monomers held together by a joining chain. It has the capacity to bind to foreign substances and activate complement, which enhances the inflammatory response.

**Immunoglobulin.** A protein secretion of B lymphocytes and plasma cells that circulates in the bloodstream and binds specifically to foreign invaders.

**Immunosuppression.** Depression of the function of the immune system, either by disease or drug treatment.

**Inflammation.** The reflexive immune response to any injury. It causes redness, swelling, heat, and pain and brings white blood cells into the area of damage to wall off germs and start the healing process.

**Inoculation.** Introduction into the body of the causative agent of a disease. Vaccinations are performed by inoculation.

**Intracellular.** Inside cells. In the sense of disease-causing germs, the ones that live inside your cells, like some bacteria, some fungi, some single-celled parasites, and all viruses.

**Killed viral vaccine.** A vaccine composed of viruses that have been treated so that they cannot infect cells.

**Killer cell.** A cell of your immune system that identifies and explodes your own tissue cells when they are infected with a disease agent or altered by cancer. They include cytotoxic T lymphocytes and natural killer cells.

**Live attenuated vaccine.** A vaccine composed of viruses that have been altered so that they complete their life cycle in the human without causing significant disease.

**Lymph node.** A secondary lymphoid organ designed to filter invaders from the extracellular spaces.

**Lymphocyte.** The category of white blood cells that control the acquired immune response. They are not phagocytic, but have subtypes that either produce antibodies, regulate the actions of other white blood cells, or kill infected cells.

**Lymphoid progenitor cell.** The stem cell found in the bone marrow that is the precursor of natural killer cells, B lymphocytes, T lymphocytes, and plasma cells.

**Lysosome.** A package of acids and digestive enzymes inside a phagocytic cell that assist in the process of intracellular digestion.

**Macrophage.** A phagocytic cell found in the tissues, which originates from a monocyte in the bloodstream. Macrophages are the cells that present proteins to T lymphocytes for specific immune recognition.

**Major histocompatibility complex (MHC).** The set of genes that encode surface molecules on each of your cells and identify your parentage. They come in two varieties, class I and class II, and serve as recognition molecules so that your immune cells can identify the cells of your body in health and in sickness.

**Mast cell.** The end cell of basophil differentiation, responsible for dumping toxic chemicals on parasites that try to get into your body. When misdirected, mast cells also cause the symptoms and signs of allergic hypersensitivity.

**Memory cell.** A cell of B or T lymphocyte lineage that has been exposed to a foreign substance, has mounted at least one response to that material, and now has become long-lived and quiescent.

**Methicillin-resistant *Staphylococcus aureus* (MRSA).** A recently emerging variant of a normal skin flora organism, *Staphylococcus aureus*, which cannot be killed with the drug methicillin.

**Monocyte.** A type of white blood cell that is phagocytic and differentiates into a tissue macrophage when it is called out of the circulation in response to inflammation.

**Monomer.** A molecule made of a single unit, as in antibodies when there is a single Y-shaped unit. IgG and IgE are monomers, whereas IgA and IgM are multimeric molecules.

**Mucosa.** The specialized linings of tissues such as the lungs, digestive organs, and excretory and genital systems that secrete mucus and prevent the entrance of germs in this way.

**Mutation.** An accidental random change in the coding of DNA that changes the molecules that an organism or cell is capable of making.

**Myeloid progenitor cell.** The bone marrow stem cell responsible for the production of red blood cells, platelets, phagocytes, and granulocytes of your body.

**Natural killer cell.** A cell of the lymphoid type related to B and T lymphocytes, but which appears to function in the absence of training in the thymus, wears surface molecules distinct from these types of lymphocytes, and functions in the control of some virus infections and some cancers.

**Natural selection.** "Survival of the fittest," the fundamental concept of evolution. The theory, originally proposed by Charles Darwin, that populations of reproducing organisms change over time when genetic traits give them an advantage or disadvantage over their competitors for space and resources. Those with advantages contribute a greater genetic input into the future generations, and those with disadvantages die out and contribute less, so that advantageous traits are selected for the future.

**Neutrophil.** A category of granulocytic white blood cells that is the most important phagocyte of your body. They are the major defense mechanism against extracellular bacteria and fungi because they eat these invaders and begin the process of abscess formation to stop germ penetration further into your body.

**Normal flora.** The bacteria and fungi that naturally live on your body surfaces (both internal and external) and contribute to your health. They may cause disease if they invade more deeply into your body or if you become immunologically challenged.

**Opsonize (opsonization).** To coat with antibody or complement fragments to speed the process of engulfment of particles by phagocytes.

**Parasite.** In its broadest sense, any organism that obtains the materials it needs for life from other organisms at their expense. In the narrow sense, an organism that is either a protozoan (single-celled parasite) or helminth (worm parasite) that lives at the expense of its host and is incapable of independent existence.

**Passive immunity.** Immunity donated from one individual to another, as in maternal transfer of antibodies across the placenta to a fetus.

**Pathogen/pathogenic.** An organism that causes disease.

**Phagocyte (phagocytosis).** A cell that ingests particles and digests them intracellularly.

**Phagocytosis.** The process of ingesting particles and digesting them.

**Plasma cell.** The end cell of B lymphocyte differentiation; the cell that is a factory for antibody production.

**Plasmid.** A small circle of DNA that probably arose as an independent life-form and now exists inside bacteria and other cells, and imparts some important characteristics to them.

**Platelets.** Small cellular fragments that circulate in the bloodstream and assist in blood clotting.

**Pneumovac.** The vaccine against *Streptococcus pneumoniae*, an important cause of meningitis and pneumonia.

**Primary immune response.** The immune response to an invader the first time it enters the body.

**Primary lymphoid organ.** The bone marrow and thymus, organs in which lymphocytes arise and receive their earliest training.

**Prophylaxis.** A medical treatment, such as a vaccine, that prevents an infectious condition; prevention of disease.

**Pseudopodia.** Literally, false feet. The cytoplasmic arms of a phagocyte that extend around a particle to engulf it.

**Red blood cell.** The cells of the circulation that carry oxygen to the tissues.

**RNA.** Ribonucleic acid; the strand of nucleic acid material used on cellular organelles called ribosomes to create protein. In our cells, DNA, which is kept in our cellular nuclei, is the main genetic code, which is transcribed into RNA form and then translated into the final protein product needed by the cell.

**Secondary immune response.** The immune response that results when memory cells (created during a primary immune response) recognize a foreign invader for a second time, and multiply wildly to dispose of it.

**Secondary lymphoid organs.** The lymph nodes and spleen; organs in which lymphocytes are exposed to foreign materials so that they can mount an immune response.

**Selection pressure.** The incentive for organisms to change their form (mutate) to survive in a hostile environment.

**Spleen.** The secondary lymphoid organ; it filters invading organisms out of the bloodstream.

**Stem cell.** A primitive cell that has the capacity to differentiate into a large number of different types of cells in the adult.

**T cell.** A lymphocyte that receives its training in the thymus and circulates to regulate immune responses (a helper) or kill infected cells (a killer).

**T helper 1 (Th1) cell.** The helper T lymphocyte that regulates the cell-mediated immune response against intracellular germs.

**T helper 2 (Th2) cell.** The helper T lymphocyte that regulates the antibody response against extracellular germs.

**Thymus.** The primary lymphoid organ, which trains T lymphocyte precursors; a bilobed organ in the chest cavity of a child.

**Toxoid.** An inactivated toxin incapable of causing disease but still able to evoke an immune response.

**Vaccination.** The inoculation of a material into an individual in order to stimulate the development of immunity against a disease agent.

**Vancomycin-resistant *Staphylococcus aureus* (VRSA).** A new variant of a normal skin flora organism, *Staphylococcus aureus*, that cannot be killed with any of the standard drugs used in hospitals, including vancomycin.

**Variable domains.** The unique ends of an antibody molecule that bind to a specific foreign substance.

**Viral load.** The amount of virus found in a patient. In HIV/AIDS it is used as a measure of the progression of disease.

**Virus.** A type of disease agent that invades your cells and depends upon them for completion of its life cycle.

**White blood cell.** One of several types of cells found in the circulation that patrol your body and protect you from invasion by germs.

# About the Author

Mary Ruebush, PhD, is a microbiology and immunology instructor for COMPASS Medical Education Network/Kaplan Medical. Her studies on germs and bacteria have been published in scholarly journals. She is the mother of two children, a daughter and a son. She lives in Bozeman, Montana.